THE COMPLETE FAMILY MEDICAL ADVISER

THE COMPLETE FAMILY MEDICAL ADVISER

Edited by:
Dr. Martin Edwards

foulsham
LONDON • NEW YORK • TORONTO • SYDNEY

foulsham
Yeovil Road, Slough, Berkshire, SL1 4JH

ISBN 0-572-01995-5

This modernised and anglicised edition
copyright © 1994 W. Foulsham Ltd.

Original copyright © Publications International Ltd.

NOTICE

In this book, the authors and editors have done their best to outline the indicated
general treatment for various conditions, diseases, ailments, and their symptoms.
Also, recommendations are made regarding certain drugs, medications and
preparations.

Different people react to the same treatment, medication, or preparation in
different ways. This book does not purport to answer all questions about all
situations that you or your family may encounter. It does not attempt to replace
your physician.

Neither the editors nor the publishers of this book take responsibility for any
possible consequences from any treatment, action or application of any
medication or preparation to any person reading or following the information or
advice contained in this book. The publication of this book does not constitute the
practice of medicine. The author and publisher advice that you consult your
physician before administering any medication or undertaking any course of
treatment.

Phototypeset in Great Britain by ROM-Data Corporation Ltd, Falmouth, Cornwall
Printed in Great Britain by St Edmundsbury Press Ltd, Bury St Edmunds, Suffolk.

Contents

Introduction

The person with the greatest influence on your own and your family's health, is you. You are the one to decide what you will eat and drink, whether to smoke or use alcohol, whether to take regular exercise.

But the decisions you take need to be based on a firm understanding of the way your body works, in health and disease.

The Complete Family Medical Adviser is not a substitute for the advice your doctor can give. It doesn't aim to show you how to diagnose and treat every illness that your family might encounter. But it does provide a great deal of clear understanding about the workings of your body, and tells you what is happening when things go wrong.

You can use this information to help plan a healthy lifestyle that suits you. You will be better able to understand and communicate with your doctor when you or your family do need to see him or her. And you will feel more confident in dealing with illness in the family.

The Complete Family Medical Adviser offers facts and explanations about the human body. The book is divided into chapters based on systems of the body (for example, the digestive system). Each chapter covers diseases, disorders, conditions, syndromes, diagnostic procedures, treatments, and medical terms pertaining to that body system. Preceding these individual entries is an introduction to the body system – a description of its parts and of how the system as a whole normally functions in a healthy body. These introductions give you a reference point for becoming familiar with the way your body should work; to understand disease as a departure from the normal healthy state of an organ or system, you should understand what is normal and healthy.

In those entries that discuss a disease or disorder, the description of the problem, the cause (if known), the symptoms, the treatment, the prognosis, and the risk factors are discussed. In addition, preventive action is outlined, if appropriate or possible. In those entries that define a term or discuss a procedure, the explanation includes examples to illustrate the concept or idea. In short, each entry attempts to be as inclusive as possible without being technical and hard to understand.

Maintaining good health is a team effort between you, your doctor, and the other members of your family who need medical care. Remember, however, that the final responsibility for your health is yours. The best way to help yourself and your family is to be informed about your medical needs. You can gain that knowledge by reading *The Complete Family Medical Adviser.*

Facts about Infectious Diseases

The human body is both surrounded by and inhabited by many living organisms. Most are so small that they are invisible to the naked eye. For this reason, they are called *micro-organisms*. Many micro-organisms are harmless or even beneficial; for example, certain bacteria that normally live in the digestive system help digest food. Occasionally, however, a micro-organism capable of causing a disease invades the body. Diseases caused by such micro-organisms are called infectious diseases.

Infectious diseases are contagious; that is, they can be passed from one person to another. They can be transmitted by skin contact, by contaminated food or drink, or by airborne particles containing the micro-organisms. Animal or insect bites are another means of transmission. (If an insect, for example, bites an infected person, the insect can pick up the micro-organism and pass the disease by biting another person.)

The two most common types of infectious diseases are bacterial infections and viral infections.

Bacteria are one-celled microscopic organisms. They normally exist in the body by the billions. Most are harmless; some, like those in the digestive tract, perform useful functions. On the other hand, some bacteria are disease-causing, or pathogenic. Disease-causing bacteria either (1) attack the body's tissues directly or (2) cause damage by secreting poisonous substances called toxins.

Fortunately, bacterial infections are frequently curable; certain bacteria can be killed by drugs called antibiotics. Other bacterial diseases can be prevented by vaccination. (Bacteria will be discussed later in this chapter.)

A virus is the smallest known micro-organism. Viruses are responsible for diseases as prevalent and relatively harmless as the common cold as well as serious diseases such as some forms of meningitis. Viruses live and reproduce only within living cells, and only certain cells are susceptible to a specific virus. You may be host to many viruses without suffering any adverse effects, but if enough cells are attacked, you may become sick.

There is no effective medical treatment for most viral infections. Because a virus lives inside a cell, any treatment designed to kill the virus is also likely to harm the cell. In addition, there are thousands of different viruses – each with different properties – and an agent effective against one virus probably will not affect the others. Although there are vaccinations for some viral diseases, therapy for most viral diseases is limited to treating the symptoms.

THE BODY'S DEFENCES

Despite the prevalence of disease-causing micro-organisms, your body is not defenceless against these invaders. The body fights infections in three ways: by preventing these organisms from entering the body; by attacking those that do manage to enter; and by inactivating those organisms it cannot kill. Sometimes, too, the body fights disease by developing defensive symptoms. Fever is an example. During an illness, the body's temperature regulator may respond to the illness by raising the body's temperature. It is thought that the micro-organism causing the disease may not be able to survive the higher body temperature.

The skin is the first barrier that guards the underlying tissues of the body. Additional protection is offered by sweat, which contains antiseptic (germ-killing) substances. Where there are natural openings in the skin, there are also defences. For example, tear glands in the eyes secrete and bathe the eyes with fluid that contains bacteria-fighting properties. The saliva glands in the mouth and the tonsils in the throat help prevent micro-organisms from attacking the mouth and throat. Many openings in the body as well as internal passages are lined with mucous membranes. These delicate layers

produce mucus, a slippery secretion that moistens and protects by repelling or trapping micro-organisms.

Internally, certain body organs fight infection. For instance,
the liver and the spleen (a large gland-like organ located in
the abdomen) filter out harmful substances from the blood
flowing through them. The lining of the stomach produces
acids that attack germs in food that has been eaten. And the

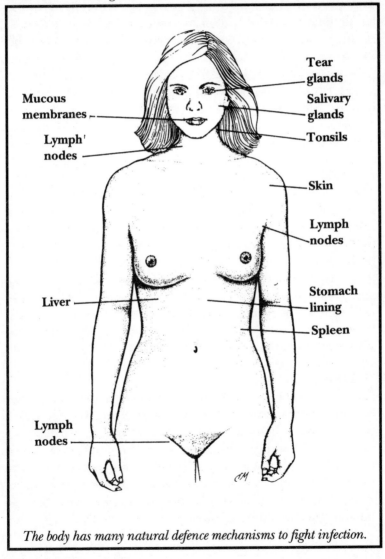

The body has many natural defence mechanisms to fight infection.

body's lymph system manufactures white blood cells whose job it is to attack and kill invading organisms.

THE LYMPH SYSTEM

The lymph system is a network of vessels that carries lymph, a watery fluid, throughout the body. Lymph drains from the blood vessels and body tissues, carrying away waste products. The waste products, including germs, are filtered out of the lymph by small glands called lymph nodes. Within the lymph nodes, unwanted micro-organisms are trapped, attacked, and destroyed by white blood cells. This is one of the body's primary and most efficient lines of defence.

The lymph system also manufactures antibodies. Antibodies are protective substances that the body produces in response to an invasion of a hostile organism. Antibodies counteract invading bacteria or viruses by inactivating them so that they are powerless. Antibodies that neutralise toxins (poisons) produced by bacteria are called antitoxins.

The body's production of white blood cells and antibodies in response to an invading disease organism is called the immune reaction. Immunity is the body's ability to resist an invasion of disease-causing bacteria and viruses. Once antibodies have been made to fight a certain micro-organism, that germ no longer poses a threat to the body. That is why one attack of a disease often prevents that same disease from infecting the body again. The first attack causes antibodies to be produced, and these antibodies protect the system against subsequent attacks.

IMMUNISATION

Immunity can also be provided artificially. This is the underlying basis of immunisation or vaccination. A vaccine is a preparation containing the offending organism – usually in a weakened form that will not cause the actual disease. When introduced into the body, the vaccine stimulates the body to produce antibodies against the disease. These antibodies remain in the system for a long time (often for life), and the body is thus prepared to resist the actual disease.

MEDICATIONS

Besides vaccination, there are other measures that can be used to help the body's natural defences fight off infectious diseases. Bacterial infections can often be conquered by drugs called antibiotics. Antibiotics, too, are products of nature. They are substances produced by living micro-organisms that kill other micro-organisms. Penicillin, for example, comes from a living mould called *Penicillium*. Penicillin and drugs related to it are among the most commonly used antibiotics, along with trimethoprim, tetracycline, and erythromycin. Each of these is effective against specific diseases. Antibiotics work either by destroying bacteria or by preventing their reproduction.

Sulphonamides (or sulfa drugs) are synthetic drugs that are also effective against infections. This type of drug is often prescribed for general infections of the body or for localised infections in the urinary and intestinal tracts.

Unfortunately, these medications do not attack viruses. Viruses, therefore, account for most of the infectious illnesses today, since no effective cures have been developed. However, some viral diseases can be prevented by immunisation. There are vaccines for polio, measles, rubella (German measles), mumps, and some strains of influenza – all of which are viral diseases. Researchers are working on a vaccine for chicken pox and shingles; however, this vaccine is not yet available to the public.

Researchers are continually searching for new ways to help the body combat infectious diseases. Medical advances against these diseases have already been dramatic; not too many years ago infectious diseases were uncontrollable and thus a constant danger. The understanding and control of infections has been one of medicine's greatest accomplishments.

Disease-causing micro-organisms and the more common infectious diseases are discussed in greater detail in the following pages.

BACTERIA

Bacteria are one-celled microscopic organisms. Some exist as chains or clumps of single cells. Some of the many different kinds of bacteria cause disease in humans and animals, but many others are beneficial. Bacteria dispose of organic waste, enrich the soil, and ferment wine and beer. They help make vinegar, cheese, and yogurt. In human beings certain beneficial bacteria live in the intestine where they help digestion.

Bacteria are different from viruses in that they are able to multiply on their own outside a living cell whereas viruses can grow and multiply only in living cells. Bacteria are different from two other causes of infection – protozoa (one-celled animals) and fungi (plant-like organisms) – in two ways: they have a primitive nucleus (centre where their genetic material is kept) rather than a well-defined one with an enclosing membrane and chromosomes; and they reproduce simply by splitting in two, as opposed to reproducing by means of a complex process (mitosis) in which their genetic material is duplicated prior to splitting.

CHICKEN POX

Chicken pox is an extremely contagious disease that is characterised by a blistery rash. It occurs most frequently in children between the ages of five and eight, and less than 20 per cent of cases occur in people over 15. Chicken pox is transmitted so easily that almost everyone gets the disease at some time.

Chicken pox is caused by infection with the virus varicella zoster. The virus creates symptoms that can be mild or severe depending upon the infected person's age.

Anyone can contract chicken pox by touching either an infected person's blisters or anything that is contaminated by them. Chicken pox is also thought to be airborne since it may be caught from an infected person before the rash develops. Yet, some researchers contend that one or two spots from the disease may be present before the rash is recognised on the body. Another way to get chicken pox is by exposure to shingles, which is a nerve disorder caused by the same virus. The incubation period for chicken pox – the time between being exposed to the illness and actually showing symptoms – is 10 to 21 days. Chicken pox is contagious until all the scabs have dried, which is usually about six to ten days after the rash appears.

SYMPTOMS
The first symptom of chicken pox is usually a rash that can be very itchy. It begins as small, red spots on the trunk. Within hours, the spots become larger, fluid-filled blisters and begin spreading out from the trunk to the face, scalp, arms, and legs. Over the next few days, the blisters continue to fill with pus, burst, and then form a scab or crust. New spots appear periodically during a two- to six-day period. They may occasionally spread to the soles and palms. The rash may even affect the eyes, mouth, throat, vagina, and rectum.

Another main symptom is a mild fever (38.5°C to 39.5°C) that rises and disappears as the rash comes and goes. Some children have a slight fever and feel sluggish a few days before the rash begins. However, this warning is more common in adults. Adults usually have higher fevers, a more severe rash, headaches and muscle aches, and they take longer to recuperate than children. Recovery from all symptoms takes ten days to two weeks.

COMPLICATIONS
Complications with chicken pox seldom develop in otherwise healthy people. The most common complication is infection of the blisters. The blister is scratched, and bacteria enter where the skin breaks. In some instances, the rash spreads to the eyes and causes pain and possible damage. Generally, the chicken pox rash heals without leaving scars unless scratched or infected. A doctor should be consulted if breathing problems,

high fever, extreme drowsiness, severe headache, vomiting, or unsteadiness occur within the course of the disease or within several weeks of recovery. These symptoms may indicate further complications such as encephalitis, an inflammation of the brain.

TREATMENT

Since there is no known cure for chicken pox, treatment constitutes reducing the effects of the symptoms. A soothing lotion, such as calamine lotion, lessens itchiness. Baths in warm (not hot) water keep the skin clean and reduce risk of infection in the rash. Baths also destroy virus in water, thereby controlling spread of the rash. If itching is severe, fingernails should be trimmed and gloves worn at night to minimise unconscious scratching. Children may need to wear gloves all day for the duration of the rash.

Junior paracetamol tablets or syrup will help to control pain

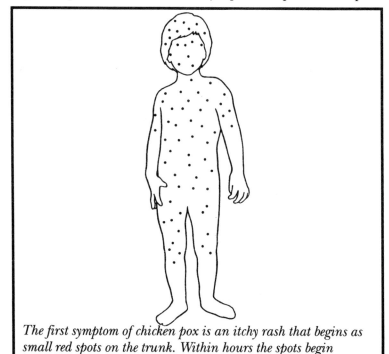

The first symptom of chicken pox is an itchy rash that begins as small red spots on the trunk. Within hours the spots begin spreading out from the trunk to the face, scalp, arms, and legs.

and fever. Aspirin isn't used for children under 12 in this country because of the possible risk of a rare but serious condition called Reye's syndrome.

Antihistamine syrup such as promethazine will help itching. Acyclovir, an anti-viral drug, can sometimes shorten chicken pox if it is given early in the disease but it is new, expensive and at present usually reserved for special cases.

PREVENTION
Researchers are trying to develop a vaccine to prevent chicken pox, but there is nothing available as yet. Although almost everyone contracts the disease once, most people do not get it again. The same organism that causes chicken pox causes the body to manufacture antibodies to combat the virus. Antibodies prevent the disease from recurring. Nevertheless, the same virus may cause shingles later in life. Why shingles occurs in some people many years after they have had chicken pox is not understood.

GONORRHOEA

Gonorrhoea is the second most frequently reported sexually transmitted, or venereal, disease in this country. It is a highly contagious infection spread primarily through direct sexual contact. The commonest sexually transmitted disease is non-specific urethritis, caused by an organism called chlamydia.

Gonorrhoea predominantly affects the penis in men, the vagina in women, and the throat and anus (opening from the intestine to the outside) in both sexes. Left untreated, it can lead to a generalised blood infection, sterility (inability to conceive children), arthritis, and heart trouble. Additionally, in men it can spread throughout the prostate gland and the male duct system, causing painful inflammation.

Gonorrhoea can also lead to eye infections if the eyes come in contact with the genital secretions – for instance, if the person rubs the eyes after handling the infected genital organs. Moreover, during the birth process, a baby may pick up eye infection from the mother's vagina if she is affected too.

CAUSES
Gonorrhoea is caused by a bacterial infection and is spread by direct sexual contact with an infected person.

SYMPTOMS
In females, this disease may exist entirely without symptoms, but in many cases it is marked by a discharge from the vagina and urethra; frequent, painful urination; cloudy urine; vomiting; and diarrhoea. Gonorrhoea often leads to pelvic inflammatory disease (PID), which, in turn, often causes sterility. (PID results when an infection in the lower reproductive or urinary tract moves to the fallopian tubes, forming scar tissue and blocking the tubes, thereby preventing conception. Its symptoms are lower abdominal pain, fever, chills and vaginal discharge.)

The symptoms of gonorrhoea in men are a yellowish

discharge from the penis within two to ten days of exposure to the disease, accompanied by painful and burning urination.

Gonorrhoea of the anus is marked by an often bloody or mucus-filled discharge from the anus and pain during bowel movements. Gonorrhoea of the throat may have no noticeable symptoms or may reveal itself only by a scratchy, sore throat.

DIAGNOSIS

Diagnosis is accomplished by taking a swab (sample) of the discharge, examining it under a microscope to identify the gonorrhoea bacterium, and confirming the diagnosis with a culture of the swab (a technique in which the sample is placed in a special substance that encourages the growth of bacteria).

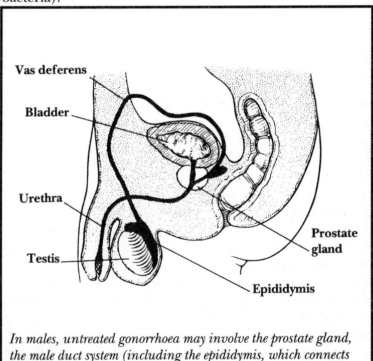

In males, untreated gonorrhoea may involve the prostate gland, the male duct system (including the epididymis, which connects the testis to the vas deferens, and the vas deferens, which conducts the sperm cells to the urethra), the bladder, and the urethra.

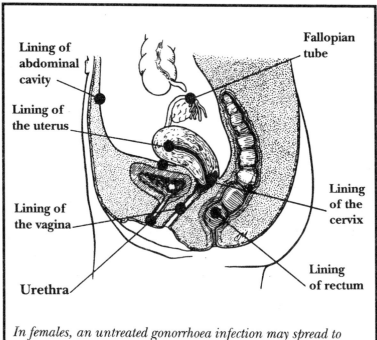

Lining of abdominal cavity

Fallopian tube

Lining of the uterus

Lining of the vagina

Lining of the cervix

Urethra

Lining of rectum

In females, an untreated gonorrhoea infection may spread to various sites in the pelvic area, as shown, causing pelvic inflammatory disease and perhaps sterility.

TREATMENT

Gonorrhoea is usually treated with penicillin, either injected or taken orally. A synthetic antibiotic is prescribed for those who are allergic to penicillin or who have contracted a penicillin-resistant strain of gonorrhoea.

While under treatment, the patient should abstain from sexual activity until further tests have confirmed that gonorrhoea is no longer present. This is usually done one week after treatment begins and sometimes again two weeks later. If signs of the disease are still present, drug therapy can be reinstated with the same antibiotic at higher dosages or perhaps with a different antibiotic.

Another sexually transmitted disease called nonspecific urethritis (NSU) sometimes occurs simultaneously with gonorrhoea, but NSU is not affected by penicillin. So if symptoms persist after regular treatment for gonorrhoea, it may be that the gonorrhoea is cleared up but NSU also is present and should be treated with another antibiotic, often tetracycline. Nowadays, special swabs and culture techniques can identify the chlamydia organism to confirm the diagnosis of NSU.

Treatment of gonorrhoea, as well as of all forms of sexually transmitted disease, requires that every sexual partner of the infected person also be examined and treated if necessary. In addition, men being treated for gonorrhoea should avoid alcoholic beverages, as it has been recently shown that drinking may increase the chance of developing an inflammation of the urethra.

PREVENTION

Gonorrhoea can be prevented, obviously, by avoiding sexual contact with someone who has the disease. However, since this is not always possible, it should be remembered that the chances of contracting the disease increase with the number of different sexual partners a person has, so limiting the number of partners may be beneficial in preventing gonorrhoea as well as other sexually transmitted diseases. Using a condom will help to stop the transmission of most sexually transmitted diseases including gonorrhoea.

HERPES

Herpes is a sexually transmitted disease, perhaps even more widespread than gonorrhoea. A sexually transmitted disease, also known as venereal disease, is a highly contagious illness spread primarily through direct sexual contact.

Herpes can be treated but not cured. Its symptoms appear briefly, then disappear, and the disease lies dormant in the nerve cells until it is reactivated by stress or illness. It is contagious only during these active periods. Persons taking drugs that suppress the body's immune system (for instance, cancer or organ transplant patients) are at a higher risk of developing herpes because their bodies are in a weakened state. There is also some evidence that links herpes with a higher rate of cancer of the cervix in women.

Although herpes is spread primarily by direct sexual contact, it can also be transmitted to an infant during childbirth, causing brain damage or death. Thus, if a woman shows signs of the active disease while in labour, the baby will be delivered by caesarian section (delivery through a surgical incision in the walls of the uterus and abdomen) rather than through the vagina where the herpes blisters may be present.

CAUSE
Herpes is caused by an infection with the herpes simplex type 2 virus which is the same kind of virus as the one that causes cold sores on the lips.

SYMPTOMS
The predominant symptom of herpes is the outbreak of painful, itching blisters filled with fluid on and around the external sexual organs. Females may have a vaginal discharge. Symptoms vaguely similar to those of the flu may accompany these outbreaks, including fever and fatigue.

The blisters will disappear without treatment in about two to ten days, but the virus will remain, lying dormant among clusters of nerve cells until another outbreak is triggered by stress, a cold, fever, or, in women, menstruation. Many patients can anticipate an outbreak by a warning sign, a tingling sensation called a 'prodrome' of the approaching illness. Herpes is contagious only during actual outbreaks, so sexual activity should be avoided while symptoms are present.

DIAGNOSIS
Diagnosis of herpes is confirmed by microscopic examination and culture of the fluid contained in the blisters.

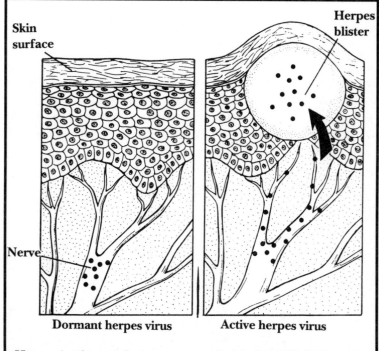

Hepres simplex type 2 virus causes painful, fluid-filled blisters in its active stage. The blisters eventually disappear, but the herpes virus lies dormant within nerve cells until stress or illness reactivate the virus, triggering a new outbreak of active herpes blisters.

TREATMENT

Herpes cannot be cured as can other sexually transmitted diseases, because any medication that will attack the virus while it lies dormant in the nerve cells will also damage the nerve cells. However, there is treatment for acute outbreaks now available that involves the use of either the antiviral drug acyclovir or laser therapy, both of which will heal blisters, reduce pain, and most importantly, kill large numbers of the herpes virus. It should be noted, however, that to be effective, therapy must be started immediately after the first sores appear and preferably even earlier, in the prodrome phase of tingling. In addition, herpes, as well as all forms of sexually transmitted disease, requires that every sexual partner of the infected person be examined and treated if necessary.

PREVENTION

Herpes can be prevented, obviously, by avoiding sexual contact with an infected person whose disease is in its active period. It should be remembered that the chances of contracting this or any other sexually transmitted disease increase with the number of different sexual partners a person has. Therefore, limiting the number of partners and using condoms can help to prevent herpes.

INFECTIOUS MONONUCLEOSIS

Infectious mononucleosis, or glandular fever, is a contagious viral disease that initially attacks the lymph glands in the neck and the throat. When these glands, which normally manufacture white blood cells that fight invading organisms, are weakened, sore throat, swollen glands and fever result.

Glandular fever is caused by a virus named Epstein-Barr virus after the scientists that first identified it in the mid-1960s. The virus enters the lymph glands and attacks the lymphocytes, the white blood cells manufactured in the lymph glands. As the white blood cells come into contact with the virus, they change shape and multiply. At first there are no symptoms, because it takes several weeks before enough of the altered cells can accumulate to generate a reaction. Gradually, however, symptoms appear. First, there is a mild sore throat, sluggishness, and fever. The symptoms worsen as the body tries to fight the infection by creating more white blood cells. Finally, symptoms diminish and disappear after about six to eight weeks.

Glandular fever spreads by contact with moisture from the mouth and throat of the infected person. Kissing, sharing drinking glasses and toothbrushes, or touching anything that has been near the mouth of an infected person transmits the disease.

Teenagers and young adults seem most susceptible. Children may become infected, but glandular fever seldom affects anyone over 35.

SYMPTOMS

Usually, the infection develops so slowly with such mild symptoms that it may be initially indistinguishable from a cold or the flu. However, a sore throat that lasts two weeks or more; swollen glands around the neck, throat, armpit, and groin; a persistent fever (usually about 39°C); and tiredness; may suggest glandular fever. The symptoms can be mild or so severe that throat pain can impede swallowing and fever may reach 40.5°C. Some people also experience a rash, eye pain, or discomfort in bright light (photophobia).

COMPLICATIONS

Glandular fever usually runs an uncomplicated course. Occasionally, however, the infection spreads to other parts of the body besides the throat and lymph glands. For example, it may lead to hepatitis, an infection of the liver. Jaundice, a symptom of this complication, appears as a yellow discoloration of the skin and whites of the eyes. Another sign the infection has travelled is pain or tenderness in the abdomen. This discomfort may mean a swollen spleen (part of the lymph system) that very rarely may rupture or burst. Any of these symptoms should be reported to a doctor for immediate attention.

DIAGNOSIS

When diagnosing infectious mononucleosis, a doctor takes a blood test. This determines if there is an excessive number of white blood cells, whether they are abnormally shaped because of the virus, and if the body is making antibodies (protective substances) to fight the Epstein-Barr virus. If it confirms that glandular fever is present the doctor may take a second blood test two weeks later, to show whether the white blood cell count is still high, indicating disease is present.

TREATMENT

Once glandular fever is confirmed, standard treatment for its symptoms is prescribed. Antibiotics are ineffective since the disease is caused by a virus that does not respond to antibiotics. As long as there are no complications, the best treatment is to stay in bed, drink plenty of liquids until the temperature returns to normal, and then gradually resume normal activities as strength returns. Aspirin or paracetamol will help pain and fever.

Antibiotics may be indicated if a bacterial infection develops in addition to glandular fever because bacteria do respond to antibiotics. In severe cases, corticosteroid drugs that reduce swelling are prescribed. If the spleen is swollen, a doctor may recommend avoiding strenuous activities, such as lifting or pushing, that may cause sudden rupture of the spleen. Hospitalisation is necessary for severe complications.

Most people recover in six to eight weeks, but some cases take as long as six months for complete recovery. A tired feeling, which may include depression, is the last symptom to disappear. Glandular fever may return in a milder form of the initial infection within a few months.

INFLUENZA

Influenza, more commonly called the flu, is a contagious disease that is accompanied by respiratory problems and fever. It is an uncomfortable illness that is usually not dangerous to otherwise healthy people.

CAUSES

Two types of viruses cause influenza: influenza A and influenza B. Each type encompasses several different strains that are named for the place where they were first identified, for example, 'Hong Kong flu' and 'Russian flu'.

The unusual characteristic about flu virus is that once one strain spreads throughout a population, the virus strain changes in structure. Therefore, it becomes a new strain carrying a new form of influenza. The antibodies, or protective substances, produced by the body to combat the virus no longer work against recurrence of that virus because the virus has taken on different qualities. Scientists are generally able to predict what type of altered virus to expect each year, but about every ten years an entirely new strain appears.

Because influenza is thought to be transmitted by airborne particles from an infected person's respiratory system, large numbers of people in a community or even in a country can easily contract the disease in a relatively short period of time. Understandably, crowds encourage transmission of the flu. In addition, since flu spreads most easily where temperatures and humidity are low, most cases of influenza occur in autumn or winter months.

SYMPTOMS

Once the body is exposed to the virus, flu symptoms develop in one to three days. Some people acquire symptoms in as short a time as 18 hours. Fever, chills, headache, muscle aches, and total exhaustion can begin suddenly. Although fevers of 38°C to 40°C are more common, body temperature may rise to 41°C.

Frequently, people experience a dry cough and runny or congested nose as their initial symptoms begin to subside. These respiratory symptoms worsen and remain for three to four days. The cough, weariness and sometimes depression may persist for two weeks or more after the other symptoms disappear.

COMPLICATIONS

The most common complications result from the virus settling in parts of the respiratory system. Old people in particular are at risk from pneumonia (infection of the lungs). If the patient has extreme difficulty in breathing, blood in the coughed-up phlegm, bluish skin, or a bark-like cough, a doctor should be consulted immediately to prevent further complications.

One life-threatening complication that affects children between the ages of two and 16 years is Reye's syndrome. It is a type of inflammation of the brain (encephalitis) that is accompanied by deteriorating changes in the liver.

TREATMENT

Influenza cannot be cured, but usually only treated by relieving symptoms. However, there is an antiviral drug that is effective against influenza A virus symptoms and in some cases the disease itself. The drug can produce unpleasant side effects and doesn't seem to help everybody, so doctors prescribe it only when a patient is susceptible to additional complications.

In most cases, treatment for flu is the same as treatment for a bad cold or fever. Doctors recommend bed rest, extra fluids, and aspirin or paracetamol to reduce fever and muscle aches. Aspirin is not recommended for a child with flu and it isn't available for children under 12 in this country because of a possible association with Reye's syndrome. Paracetamol is quite safe though. Nasal sprays or drops, when used sparingly so nasal tissues are not damaged, and cough medicines help relieve cold-like symptoms. A vaporizer in the patient's room that adds moisture to the air relieves congestion.

PREVENTION

Each year, researchers prepare an influenza vaccine in an attempt to prevent spread of the virus. The vaccine is composed of several different virus strains and provides protection against influenza from these strains. Regrettably, protection is not necessarily afforded against new or different strains. Vaccines are typically between 67 and 92 per cent effective.

Some people have reactions from the vaccine that range from inflammation at the site of the injection to mild flu symptoms. Children under four wouldn't normally be given the vaccine, and older children may receive a special form of the jab to reduce the risk of any reactions.

MEASLES

Measles is a contagious disease that mainly affects the respiratory system, skin and eyes. It was once considered one of the more dangerous childhood diseases because the threat of serious complications was so great. Fortunately, development of a vaccine to prevent measles has drastically reduced its occurrence.

CAUSES

Another name for measles is rubeola. Rubeola is caused by a virus that invades the body and infects living cells. The virus comes from the respiratory system of an infected person and is spread via droplets of moisture that travel through the air. Some researchers contend that the virus enters the body through the eyes.

Incubation period for measles – the time between being exposed to the illness and actually showing symptoms – is eight to 12 days. During this time the infected person is contagious up to four days before symptoms begin and up to six days after the rash develops.

SYMPTOMS

Measles usually begins much like a cold with runny nose, nasal congestion, sneezing, a dry cough, and fever between 39°C and 40°C. After three or four days, eyes may become sensitive to bright light as they grow red and swollen. Then the fever drops. At this time, red spots with tiny white centres appear in the mouth. These are called Koplik's spots after the man who first diagnosed them.

By the fourth or fifth day, the fever increases again, and a rash appears. The rash usually starts on the face, neck, and behind the ears before spreading to the rest of the body. As the spots multiply, they grow larger, become raised, and sometimes blend together. Their colour turns dark red and then brown before the skin begins to fall off in small flakes. This process takes about one week after the rash first emerges, although skin discoloration can last as long as two weeks. Other symptoms usually disappear within seven to ten days from the start of the disease.

COMPLICATIONS

Breathing problems, increased coughing, earache, or extreme drowsiness may indicate complications that warrant consulting a doctor immediately. The more serious complications are pneumonia (infection of the lungs) and encephalitis (inflammation of the brain). Additionally, sub-acute sclerosing panencephalitis (SSPE), a rare but often fatal disease of the brain, has been linked to measles. Severe ear infections can also result, particularly in young children. In addition, bronchitis, laryngitis, and swollen neck glands can complicate measles and make the course of the illness last longer or even return after apparent recovery.

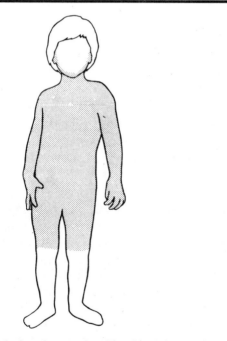

The measles rash – dark red spots that blend together as they spread – usually begins on the face, neck, and behind the ears and then spreads over the body as far as the knees.

DIAGNOSIS

Generally, doctors diagnose measles by the initial symptoms. To confirm diagnosis, nasal discharge, blood, or urine can be tested for signs of the virus.

TREATMENT

Measles, being caused by a virus, does not respond to antibiotics. For this reason, treatment focuses upon relieving uncomfortable symptoms. A vaporizer in the patient's room eases cold-like symptoms by adding moisture to the air. If the eyes are irritated, warm compresses may relieve the inflammation. Also, dim lights are easier on the eyes. When washing, soaps that may irritate the skin should not be used. A doctor may suggest adding baking soda to bath water or applying a soothing lotion, such as calamine lotion, to the rash to relieve itching. Most doctors recommend paracetamol to reduce fever.

PREVENTION

Today, measles is much less common because of a vaccine given to children as an injection between 12 and 15 months of age. The vaccine, which is prepared from measles virus, stimulates antibody (protective substance in cells) action within the body to produce immunity or resistance to the disease. It is given together with vaccination against mumps and rubella (German measles) as the combined MMR vaccine. A low vaccine effectiveness rate in very young children is the reason that babies are not vaccinated before 12 months of age. Most babies under six months of age already have immunity that they acquired from their mothers before birth. Should a baby be exposed to measles, however, a doctor should be consulted. Measles is dangerous for anyone under three years of age or for anyone with chronic (long-term) disease.

MUMPS

Mumps is a highly contagious viral disease that is usually contracted during childhood. More than 85 per cent of the cases occur before age 15, especially between six and ten years of age.

CAUSE

Mumps is caused by a virus that attacks cells of the salivary glands. Usually it affects the parotid salivary glands, causing painful swelling of the face beneath the ear along the jawline. Mumps virus spreads by contact with airborne moisture from the infected person's nose or throat. Sometimes, the infection comes from someone who either has the disease without symptoms or who is not yet aware of the symptoms. The disease occurs most often during spring months, though it can happen any time of year.

SYMPTOMS

Symptoms can be so mild that they are nonexistent or they can be very severe. Fever (38.5°C to 39.5°C), headache, and loss of appetite usually develop first, followed by earache. Then the characteristic swelling of the salivary glands appears. Swelling may start on one side of the face and then appear on the other side within a few days. Sometimes, however, only one side swells. The inflammation may cause soreness and difficulty in eating or swallowing.

Other glands, such as the sex glands, or other salivary glands under the jaw, may become swollen as well. Boys who have one or both testes inflamed may be in considerable pain. The affected testicle may shrink somewhat, but it always returns to normal size in time. Medically, this condition is known as orchitis. Contrary to popular belief, mumps uncommonly leads to sterility in males. Girls may have swelling in the ovaries (female sex organs), but there is seldom any severe discomfort. In addition, swelling may occur in other glands and organs including the breasts, other salivary glands, liver and the brain.

COMPLICATIONS

Although mumps can be unpleasant, it rarely has long-term complications. If they do occur, encephalitis (inflammation of the brain) is the most dangerous complication of mumps because it carries the risk of death. Another possible result of mumps encephalitis is hearing loss or even deafness. However, hearing may return to normal after several months. A milder form of brain complication is meningoencephalitis (inflammation of the brain or its covering, the meninges). This disease causes stiff neck, headache, high fever, drowsiness, bright light sensitivity, and possible delirium – all symptoms that usually disappear without damage to the brain.

Pancreatitis, or inflammation of the pancreas, can also result from mumps. Symptoms of this complication are stomach pain, vomiting, chills, fever, and extreme weakness. Although these signs usually vanish and leave no damage, diabetes can result in rare cases. Other complications of mumps include nerve inflammation, heart problems, and nervous system disorders – all usually temporary.

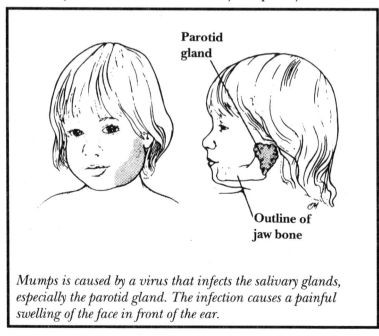

Parotid gland

Outline of jaw bone

Mumps is caused by a virus that infects the salivary glands, especially the parotid gland. The infection causes a painful swelling of the face in front of the ear.

DIAGNOSIS

A doctor diagnoses mumps by examining the characteristic form and texture of the swollen parotid glands. Boys may have swelling and tenderness in the testes. Exposure to the disease is also a clue. Incubation – time between exposure to the virus and signs of symptoms – is 14 to 21 days. If mumps is suspected, secretions from the salivary glands can be tested for mumps virus although this isn't generally necessary.

TREATMENT

Treatment for mumps involves relieving discomfort of the symptoms, since there is no cure for the disease. Bed rest is usually not necessary. Soft foods and liquids may be easier to swallow. However, fruit juices with high acid content, like orange or grapefruit, may sting.

If glands are severely swollen, a doctor may suggest paracetamol or other painkillers. Steroid drugs may be recommended for men or boys with extremely swollen testes, but these drugs may prove ineffective. Warm or cold compresses including an ice pack may relieve some pain. Most mumps symptoms disappear within about ten days.

PREVENTION

There is a vaccine that is 95 per cent effective in preventing mumps. The vaccine encourages antibodies (protective substances) to be produced by the body to resist the disease. It is combined with measles and rubella (German measles) vaccines as the MMR vaccine, and given to children as a jab between 12 and 15 months.

RUBELLA

Rubella, or German measles, is a relatively mild viral infection with cold-like symptoms and a short-lived rash. The disease is contagious, but it is usually not dangerous. One exception is when rubella infects pregnant women. In this instance, the virus can also affect the unborn child, causing serious long-term problems. However, rubella outbreaks are infrequent since the development of a vaccine to prevent the illness.

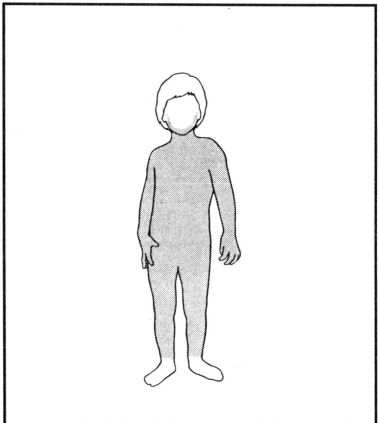

The light pink rubella rash first appears on the face and the neck and then gradually spreads over most of the body.

CAUSE

Rubella results from a virus that invades the cells of the body. The virus spreads from one person to another by contact with airborne moisture from the infected person's respiratory system. An infected person can spread the virus as early as one week before the rash appears and as late as five days after the rash fades. A baby with congenital rubella syndrome can transfer the virus until the child is about 12 to 18 months old. Although instances of second infections have been reported, rubella seldom occurs twice in the same person.

SYMPTOMS

The first symptoms of rubella are runny nose, swollen neck glands, and low fever (up to 38.5°C). About two days after these signs, a rash with very small red or pink spots appears on the face and neck. The spots are flat initially. Then they become slightly raised and fade within a day or two. As the first spots fade, more spots develop until the rash gradually spreads over most of the body. The rash lasts only two to three days, but swollen glands may persist for as long as a week. All other symptoms usually disappear by then. When there is joint pain, as is common with older women, discomfort may last another week.

COMPLICATIONS

Although rubella is generally a mild infection, some complications can arise. Encephalitis, or inflammation of the brain, occurs in one in 5000 cases. Thrombocytopaenic purpura, a blood disease, can prove fatal when it accompanies rubella. High or prolonged fever and extreme fatigue should be reported to a doctor to prevent further complications.

Another serious complication of rubella is congenital rubella syndrome, or rubella infection that is present at birth. Here the pregnant woman transmits the disease to the foetus (unborn child) during pregnancy. Rubella virus may cause one or more serious organic and growth disorders, particularly if contracted during the first three months of pregnancy when the foetus is forming. The most common problems include congenital heart defects, hearing and vision problems, blood disorders, and mental retardation and other brain disorders.

DIAGNOSIS

Under normal circumstances, rubella is difficult to diagnose because the symptoms are so mild and variable. Sometimes a rash is absent and the disease resembles a cold. Other cases may be so severe that the infection may be confused with measles. A doctor can identify the virus by taking a blood test and tracing any history of exposure to the disease and this may be necessary in the case of a pregnant woman. Incubation, or time between contact with the virus and beginning of symptoms, is 14 to 21 days.

TREATMENT

Most patients require little or no treatment for rubella because the symptoms are so mild. Aspirin in adults, or paracetamol in children, may afford relief for any joint pain. Otherwise, drugs are not needed. Some patients may want bed rest, but most people feel well enough to be somewhat active.

PREVENTION

Rubella rarely occurs now because children routinely receive rubella vaccine between 12 and 15 months of age. The vaccine is combined with measles and mumps vaccine in one injection (MMR). Rubella vaccine works in the body to stimulate antibodies (protective substances) that fight the disease. Rubella vaccination used to be given only to girls around the age of 12. Now it is offered to all children between 12 and 15 months instead, as part of the combined MMR vaccine. Some schoolgirls will still need the jab at age 12 for the next few years, though, as they wouldn't have had it when they were younger – MMR wasn't introduced in this country until 1988.

Women who want to become pregnant should take a blood test to determine whether they are already immune (resistant) to the disease. If not, they too, can receive a vaccination. Vaccinations are not recommended for pregnant women because of a risk of infection to the foetus. For this reason also, doctors caution women to wait at least three months after vaccination before becoming pregnant.

SHINGLES

Shingles, or herpes zoster, is a painful viral infection of one or more nerves. The infection produces a blistery, itchy skin rash above the affected nerve.

CAUSES

Shingles rash looks identical to the rash of the chicken pox virus. Shingles and chicken pox are caused by the same virus called varicella zoster. Moreover, previous infection with chicken pox is necessary in order to develop shingles. Why shingles occurs in certain people and not others at any given time is unknown. Scientists believe that after recovery from chicken pox the varicella zoster virus lies dormant in the body. One theory contends that the virus is reactivated after injury to the affected area or other emotional or physical upset to the body. Sixty-five per cent of the cases studied confirm this assumption.

Another theory proposes that with shingles the number and strength of antibodies (protective substances) produced by the body to fight the varicella zoster virus may diminish after a bout of chicken pox. This reduction in force makes some individuals susceptible to another attack of the virus. Because some antibodies endure, the person gets shingles rather than chicken pox. Yet, if someone is exposed to the virus as an adult and has not had chicken pox, he or she will get chicken pox, not shingles.

Incidence of the disease increases with age. Shingles rarely occurs in people under age 15. More than 50 per cent of those who get shingles are over 45 years of age.

SYMPTOMS

Shingles begins with a prickling or tenderness in the skin over the infected nerve. Burning or shooting pain in the same area is also an early symptom. Within two to four days a rash with small, red spots appears over the affected part of the body. As the spots enlarge, they blister and sometimes blend together.

Eventually they fill with pus, burst, and crust over much the same as with chicken pox rash. With shingles, however, the process takes longer and is confined to the skin area above the affected nerve.

Shingles rash is very itchy. In addition, pain increases as the area beneath the rash becomes more red and swollen. Shingles attacks nerves on the chest, back, neck, arm or leg most often. However, facial nerves are involved frequently. The rash appears in a band or strip following the path of the nerve, usually on one side of the body. The rash persists two to three weeks before clearing, while the pain continues for three or four weeks. Sometimes, pain may linger for a month or more. In people over 60, pain may persist for several months after the rash disappears.

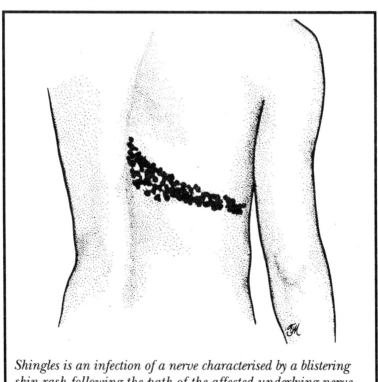

Shingles is an infection of a nerve characterised by a blistering skin rash following the path of the affected underlying nerve. The rash itself is identical to the rash of chicken pox, since both diseases are caused by the same virus.

COMPLICATIONS

Occasionally, shingles rash becomes generalised and spreads over the entire body. This develops most often in people who have underlying disease such as Hodgkin's disease (cancer of the lymph system) or leukaemia (cancer of the blood). When these serious disorders already exist, shingles can cause death, but this is rare.

The most common complication of shingles is a bacterial infection in the rash. This can prolong the rash and cause skin scars.

Less common complications follow a shingles attack on facial nerves. Eye disorders and Bell's palsy (a disease that temporarily paralyses one side of the face) can result. Shingles in other parts of the body can cause similar temporary paralysis of the area over the affected nerve.

TREATMENT

Since there is no known cure for shingles, treatment focuses on reducing pain. An analgesic, or painkilling drug, may relieve burning. Some doctors prescribe steroid drugs to reduce nerve inflammation in older patients. In order to be effective, steroids must be taken soon after shingles begins. Steroid treatment is not recommended for people with underlying disease because steroids can interfere with natural resistance to infection.

Preventing infection is also important. Baths in warm (not hot) water soothe and clean the skin. For severe itching, patients should cut their fingernails and wear gloves when asleep to control unconscious scratching. Antiviral tablets called acyclovir can help to reduce the duration of an attack of shingles provided they are taken early in the attack. They are expensive, and doctors usually reserve them for people who are very elderly or ill in some other way.

SYPHILIS

Syphilis is a serious, highly contagious disease spread primarily through direct sexual contact. Syphilis is caused by spiral-shaped bacteria called spirochaetes.

Over time, syphilis can affect all parts of the body, the brain, bones, spinal cord and heart, as well as the reproductive organs. If left untreated, blindness, brain damage, heart disease, and even death can result. Syphilis can also be passed from a mother to her unborn baby, causing congenital syphilis in the child, which may eventually result in blindness and deafness, among other serious consequences. Syphilis in a pregnant woman must be treated prior to the eighteenth week of the pregnancy in order to prevent passage of the disease to the foetus.

STAGES AND SYMPTOMS

Syphilis is a progressive disorder that passes through four stages: primary, secondary, latent, and late or tertiary. Each of the four stages of syphilis is marked by a distinct set (or lack) of symptoms.

Primary syphilis is characterised by the appearance of a painless, open sore (called a chancre) ten to 90 days after exposure to the disease. As a rule, there is usually only one sore (although occasionally there are several), appearing most commonly on the genital organs, but also at times on the rectum, cervix (the opening to the uterus), lips, tongue, fingers, or anywhere that direct contact was made. The chancre first appears as a red bump, sometimes surrounded by a red ring and oozing clear fluid; it soon erodes into a painless ulcer and disappears within several weeks without treatment. Although the chancre is gone, the disease is still active in the body.

Secondary syphilis appears within six weeks to six months of initial contact. Symptoms resembling the flu such as fever, sore throat, headache, fatigue, aching joints, and enlarged lymph nodes are common. Syphilitic meningitis (an infection of the membranes lining the brain and spinal cord) can also be seen in this stage.

Secondary syphilis is also characterised by extremely contagious, greyish-white erosions that can be seen on the lining of the mouth, the penis, the external female sexual organs, the anus, and warm, moist areas such as the underarms; by growths resembling warts in the genital area (not to be confused with the more common nonsyphilitic genital warts); and by a rash on the palms or soles in the form of round reddish spots that occur in patches and do not itch. These sores, growths and rashes heal within three to six weeks without treatment, and the disease enters the third stage.

In the latent stage (latent means present but not manifesting itself), all symptoms disappear, the patient appears to be healthy, and the disease is probably not contagious (except in the case of pregnant women, who can still pass it on to their offspring). The latent stage can go on indefinitely, but it is felt that one third of those with latent syphilis will progress to the final stage of the illness.

By the late or tertiary stage of syphilis, the disease is in all likelihood no longer contagious, but the entire body may come under siege. Late syphilis can damage the brain, bones, spinal cord and heart, commonly causing blindness, brain damage, heart disease, or even death.

DIAGNOSIS
Syphilis is diagnosed with a history and physical examination, blood tests, and a microscopic examination of a swab (sample) taken from the sores or rash areas. Several blood tests may be necessary, as the bacteria may not show up on blood tests during the first one to two weeks after exposure to the infected person.

TREATMENT
Treatment of syphilis is accomplished with the administration of penicillin, or other antibiotics if a penicillin allergy exists. Some cases of late syphilis are so advanced, however, that they will not benefit from treatment.

A person who has syphilis or any other sexually transmitted

disease should abstain from sexual activity until all tests have confirmed that the disease is no longer present. Syphilis, as well as all forms of sexually transmitted diseases, requires that every sexual partner of the infected person also be tested and treated if necessary.

PREVENTION
Syphilis can be prevented by avoiding sexual contact with someone who has the disease. However, since this is not always possible, it is important to remember that the chances of contracting this or any other sexually transmitted disease increase with the number of different sexual partners a person has, so limiting the number of partners can be beneficial to some extent in prevention. As with other sexually transmitted diseases, the regular use of condoms will cut down the rate of spread.

TETANUS

Tetanus is an acute disease of infectious origin, commonly associated with improperly cleaned deep wounds, that causes severe muscle contraction or tightening.

CAUSE
Tetanus is caused by toxins (poisonous substances) that are produced by the bacteria *Clostridium tetani.* These bacteria usually enter the body through a wound in contact with material, such as soil, in which bacteria spores are present or by being present on the skin at the time of the injury. Puncture wounds seem especially vulnerable to tetanus infection since they are, by their nature, difficult to clean and medicate, and allow little air to reach the deep tissue (these bacteria cannot live in the air).

SYMPTOMS

Tetanus symptoms are varied, depending on the extent of the infection and the body part that is affected. The most common symptom is called 'lockjaw', in which the muscles of the jaw go into severe continuous contraction, thus rendering the jaw immobile. Symptoms also include a bowed or arched body (which is rare) because of contraction of lower back muscles; back muscle spasms; and lethal throat spasms that can cause blockage of the airway. The affected body parts become immobile because of the simultaneous and continuous contraction of opposing muscles.

In severe cases, the contractions affect most of the cells in the affected muscle. The contraction is thus not merely a weak 'twitch', but is instead an almost 'complete' contraction, similar to what would be required in lifting a heavy weight or marshalling all the potential force of a muscle against a high resistance.

TREATMENT

Treatment consists of muscle relaxant drugs such as diazepam to ease the contractions. Antimicrobial drugs such as penicillin are used to fight the infection. Tetanus antitoxin is given intramuscularly in the hope of lessening the severity of the disease. However, the antitoxin does not counteract toxin already in the nervous system nor does it act to relieve symptoms already present.

PREVENTION

Immunisation beforehand with the tetanus vaccine offers the best preventive against the disease. Also, wounds should be attended to immediately, especially puncture wounds. Tetanus 'boosters' should be taken periodically, especially if small skin wounds are a common occurrence in the course of the workday. Most doctors nowadays recommend that everyone should receive a tetanus booster every 10 years.

Facts about Allergies and the Immune System

Immunity is the body's ability to defend itself against harmful substances. Essentially, it is a resistance to infection that may be inherited or acquired naturally or artificially.

Resistance occurs when foreign organisms enter the body, causing particular specialised cells to react either by attacking the organism directly or by producing proteins (compounds essential to living cells) that neutralise its effects. The most common of these organisms are forms of bacteria (one-celled organisms that have the potential to attack body tissues or secrete poisonous substances called toxins) and viruses (the smallest infective agents responsible for a variety of diseases).

LYMPH SYSTEM

The lymph system is the body's drainage system. It is composed of a network of vessels and small structures called lymph nodes. The lymph vessels carry away excess fluid collected from all over the body back into the blood circulation. Along the way, however, these fluids are forced to percolate through a lymph node so that they can be 'filtered'. Unwanted organisms are trapped and destroyed by the specialised white blood cells (lymphocytes) that are present in these nodes. Lymphocytes are also added to the lymph that flows out of nodes and back to the bloodstream.

ANTIBODIES

The lymph system also manufactures antibodies. Antibodies are specialised proteins that the body produces in response to invasion of a foreign substance called an antigen. The outer surface of an invading organism is coated with these

46

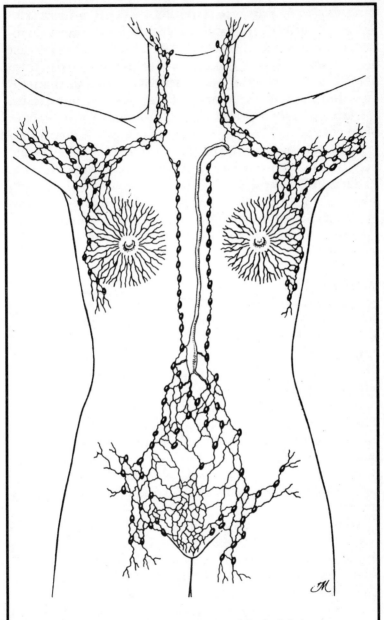

The lymph system – an important part of the body's immune system – is a network of vessels and small glands called lymph nodes whose function is to trap and destroy invading organisms.

antigens – in fact they are simply molecules of protein. The process of antibody formation begins when an antigen stimulates a lymph node into action. Antibodies then counteract invading organisms by combining with the antigens on their outer surface. Once the antibodies have coated the harmful organism, the body's scavenger cells can destroy it more easily.

During periods of active antibody production, lymph nodes often enlarge and become tender to the touch. A vaccination – or injection of a natural or artificial antigen to stimulate the body to produce protective antibodies – in the arm can cause swelling under the armpit, while an influenza infection can affect neck glands. Enlarged nodes can be felt under the skin of the armpit, groin or neck. The spleen, an organ located in the upper left part of the abdomen, is also important in the manufacture of antibodies.

IMMUNE REACTION

Production of white blood cells and antibodies in response to an invading disease organism is called an immune reaction. This immune reaction is one of the body's primary and most efficient lines of defence. Once antibodies have been produced to fight a certain organism, that germ no longer poses a threat to the body. That is why one attack of a disease often prevents that same disease from infecting the body again. The first attack causes antibody production. In turn, these antibodies protect the body against subsequent attacks. With measles, for example, the antibodies created by having the disease or by being vaccinated with measles virus resist a second attack of the disease, thus providing immunity against its recurrence.

Antibodies are not always beneficial. For example, when tissue from another body, such as a transplanted heart, is introduced, antibodies are produced to destroy the 'invader'. Transplants usually are made possible only by means of drugs and occasionally radiation that act against the body's immune response. Also, when you have a blood transfusion, it must be of a matching type; otherwise your body will manufacture antibodies to destroy it.

Sometimes, the immune system causes reactions that make

the body unusually sensitive to foreign material. When the immune response is disruptive to the body, it is called an allergic reaction.

ALLERGIC REACTION
An allergy is an extraordinary reaction or sensitivity to a particular environmental substance by the immune system.

Although it can be present almost immediately after exposure to the irritant, an allergy usually develops over time, while the immune system forms antibodies as a reaction to an invasion by a foreign substance. Under normal conditions, such antibodies work to protect the body from further attack. In the case of an allergy, however, the antibodies and other specialised cells involved in this protective function trigger an unusual sensitivity to the foreign substance (called an allergen). The antibodies then stimulate the special cells to produce histamine, a powerful chemical released from the cells that causes the small blood vessels to enlarge, the smooth muscles (such as those in the air passages or the digestive tract) to constrict, and hives (nettle rash) to develop.

No one knows why allergies develop, but it is known that an allergy can appear, disappear, or reappear at any time and at any age. Allergic reactions rarely occur during the first encounter with the troublesome allergen because the body needs time to accumulate the antibodies. Also, a family history of allergies seems to be related to an individual's sensitivity to certain allergens. People who show a tendency to develop allergies are referred to as 'atopic'. This state of atopy frequently runs in families.

An allergic reaction can be so mild that it is barely noticeable or so severe that a person's life is threatened. Common symptoms of allergy are itchy watery eyes, runny nose, itching or inflamed skin, or a swollen mouth or throat. Some allergic reactions may be accompanied by headaches, sinus stuffiness, a reduced sense of taste or smell, or difficult breathing.

An extremely severe allergic reaction, called anaphylactic shock, is characterised by breathing difficulties (caused by swelling of the throat and larynx and narrowing of the bronchial tubes), itching skin, hives, and collapse of the blood vessels, as well as by vomiting, diarrhoea, and cramps. This advanced condition can be fatal if not properly treated.

TYPES

There are four categories of allergens: inhalants, contactants, ingestants, and injectants.

Inhalant allergens are breathed in, and include such substances as dust, pollen, feathers, and animal dander (small scales from the animal's skin). Hay fever is an inhalant allergy in which the mucous membranes react to various inhaled substances, usually the pollens associated with the changing seasons. Year-round hay fever may be a reaction to pet dander, feathers, mould, or dust. Hay fever symptoms include itching of the nose, eyes, and roof of the mouth; sneezing; headache; and watery itching eyes.

Contactant allergens are those that are touched and include such substances as poison ivy, cosmetics, detergents, fabrics and dyes. Contact dermatitis is an example of an allergic-type reaction resulting from exposure to a contactant. Skin becomes inflamed, burning and itching where it has come in contact with soaps, detergents, household cleaners, drugs, or chemicals found in food or cosmetics.

Ingestant allergens are swallowed or eaten. A variety of foods and medications can act as ingestant allergens to persons overly sensitive to them. A food allergy usually occurs in children and is a reaction to an ingestant allergen, often milk, eggs, shellfish and other fish, peanuts, chocolate, strawberries, and citrus fruits. Symptoms of food allergies include abdominal cramps, nausea, vomiting, and diarrhoea. Hives, rash, headache, nasal congestion, even anaphylactic shock can also accompany a food allergy.

Injectant allergens are substances that penetrate the skin, such as insect venom or drugs that are injected. For example, people who have severe allergic reactions to insect bites or stings are suffering from a reaction to an injectant allergen. Shortness of breath; strong, rapid heartbeat; coughing; wheezing; and light-headedness; are common symptoms. The bite area swells and becomes tender or numb, and, in extreme cases, anaphylactic shock may occur.

DIAGNOSIS

In any allergy case, identifying the offending allergen may be painful, time-consuming, and expensive, but it is necessary to avoid future allergic reactions. A medical history and a record of any recent changes in daily habits are most important. Skin scratch tests (in which small amounts of the suspected allergens are applied to tiny scratches in the skin) and intracutaneous skin tests (in which allergens are injected under the skin) are also used to help detect the troublesome foreign substance. A blood test called RAST (radio-allergosorbent technique) is often taken to measure the amount of antibodies in the blood that have been manufactured in response to an invading substance.

TREATMENT

Once the allergen is pin-pointed, half the battle is won. Obviously, avoiding the troublesome allergen is a good start toward relieving an allergy problem. However, if the allergen cannot be avoided or removed, two treatments may be recommended: medication or immunotherapy. Three types of medication have commonly been prescribed: antihistamine drugs, which combat the effect of the histamines in the body; corticosteroids, which reduce inflammation and swelling; and bronchodilators, which ease breathing in asthma by opening bronchial tubes.

Allergy immunotherapy, or treatment by 'desensitisation shots', consists of the injection into the body of first small, then increasingly larger, quantities of the allergen. This allows the body to build up a form of resistance or immunity to the offending substance. It doesn't always work, and can actually be dangerous or even fatal. For this reason it is rarely used in this country, except in hospital for very severe cases.

A little common sense goes a long way in controlling allergies. Obviously, the offending allergen needs to be avoided, removed, or replaced. Natural fibres in the home can be replaced with synthetics; air conditioners or air filters can be installed for hay fever sufferers; those susceptible to insect bites can wear protective clothes, use insect repellents and avoid bright clothing and perfumes, both of which attract insects; babies born into allergy-prone families should be breast-fed as long as possible to delay exposure to cow's milk.

PREVENTION

Allergies cannot really be prevented, but much can be done to help to control or diminish their effects.

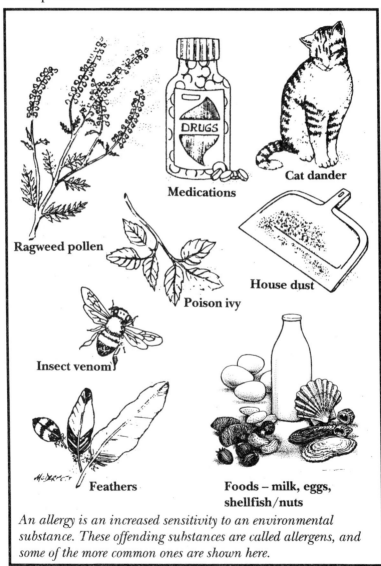

Ragweed pollen

Medications

Cat dander

Poison ivy

House dust

Insect venom

Feathers

Foods – milk, eggs, shellfish/nuts

An allergy is an increased sensitivity to an environmental substance. These offending substances are called allergens, and some of the more common ones are shown here.

AIDS – ACQUIRED IMMUNE DEFICIENCY SYNDROME

Acquired immune deficiency syndrome (AIDS) is a condition in which the body's immunity, its natural defence system against disease, is somehow severely jeopardised thus enabling organisms that are normally fought off by the body quite effectively to become deadly.

The cause of the new disease, discovered in 1979, is thought to be infection by the human immunodeficiency virus (HIV). What is known is that male homosexuals, drug addicts who inject drugs, and haemophiliacs who receive blood transfusions for their disorder are all high risk groups. Homosexual practices (for example, rectal intercourse), use of nonsterile needles within a group, possible environmental factors, and multiple transfusions of pooled blood factors have all been respectively mentioned as possible means of transmission of an agent causing the syndrome. When the disease was first reported in America, 75 per cent of victims were male homosexuals, 12 per cent intravenous drug abusers, and 0.5 per cent haemophiliacs – but 6 per cent were Haitian immigrants who were neither homosexuals nor drug abusers. But now some doctors fear that the epidemic is spreading to heterosexuals in low risk groups, emphasising the need for continuous precautions.

SYMPTOMS
Symptoms include low-grade fever, swollen lymph glands, weight loss, fatigue, night sweats, long-standing diarrhoea, and a general sick feeling. Up to one third of the victims develop a previously rare cancer known as Kaposi's sarcoma, which can appear as purplish bumps on the skin. Many come down with a severe form of pneumonia. The main problem, however, is the inability of the body to fight many diseases that

come along, including various cancers, skin infections, fungus growths, and tuberculosis.

Individuals with AIDS almost uniformly have reduced numbers of lymphocytes. These are specialised white blood cells that are critical in combating infectious diseases, particularly those caused by tuberculosis, fungi and viruses. Lymphocytes may also be instrumental in destroying malignancies in their early stages. There are two types of lymphocytes actively engaged in coping with infection: the T-cell and the B-cell. The T-cell is mainly concerned with direct cytotoxicity, that is, by a series of complex processes, it directly kills invaders. The B-cell, on the other hand, is concerned with the production of infection-fighting antibodies when stimulated. In AIDS the T-cells are greatly reduced; in fact, it is the 'helper' T-cell (a further subdivision) that is most profoundly decreased.

TREATMENT

Treatment to counter the effects of AIDS may involve the use of antibiotics, surgery to remove skin cancer, chemotherapy, and drugs to raise the body's resistance to diseases. No cure for the disease itself has been found yet although anti-viral drugs, such as zidovudine can help especially in the early stages.

Preventing AIDS means avoiding the HIV virus that causes it. Of course drug addicts shouldn't inject, but if they do they mustn't share needles. Many areas of the country offer needle exchange schemes to provide clean needles.

Condoms help to stop the spread of the virus through either homosexual or heterosexual intercourse. They are worth considering even if they aren't necessary for contraception, and should be considered essential protection in casual sex.

If you need medical treatment in countries such as most of Africa where HIV and AIDS are very common, it may be difficult to be sure whether needles are clean. Take a supply of clean needles and syringes with you – special packs are available from some chemists, doctors or travel agents.

HAY FEVER

Hay fever is a type of allergy in which the membranes of the nose react to an inhaled substance. For this reason, this substance is called an inhalant allergen.

CAUSES

Hay fever may be caused by a variety of environmental substances, but acute (short-lived), seasonal attacks are usually allergic reactions to pollen (the allergen). Most often, spring attacks are reactions to tree pollen; summer attacks are reactions to grass pollen; and autumn attacks are reactions to weed pollen. Chronic (year-round) hay fever may be an allergic reaction to a number of other substances, including pet dander (scales of dry skin on pets), certain fibres, feathers, dust and moulds.

SYMPTOMS

The symptoms of hay fever are usually the same, regardless of the allergen causing the irritation. Common symptoms include itching of the nose and roof of the mouth; a thin, watery discharge constantly draining from the nose; itchy, watery eyes; sneezing; headache; irritability; a feeling of exhaustion; insomnia; loss of appetite; and, in advanced cases where asthma is also present, coughing and wheezing.

DIAGNOSIS

Hay fever, as well as other allergies, is diagnosed by identifying the allergen. This is done by taking a medical history and reviewing the patient's environment, daily habits, and recent changes in lifestyle. Skin tests and blood tests may also be taken but aren't usually necessary. These include scratch tests, in which a small amount of the suspected allergen is applied to a scratch on the skin; intracutaneous tests, in which a small amount of the allergen is injected in or under the skin; and the radioallergosorbent technique, in which specific antibodies (developed in response to suspected allergens) in the blood are measured.

TREATMENT

A severe case of hay fever may be best treated by a change in environment, that is, removing or reducing the allergen causing the trouble. Those reacting to weed pollen may need to move to a more urban, less pollinated location; those allergic to household dusts may have to dust and wet mop more frequently; those reacting to pets or fibres in carpeting, stuffed furniture, or draperies may need to remove these allergens from the household. In addition, many hay fever sufferers would benefit from an air conditioner, which helps keep pollen and dust levels in the home to a minimum.

Several medications are available for the hay fever sufferer: oral antihistamines, which fight the histamine that is released by the body as a reaction to the forming antibodies; corticosteroids, which reduce swelling; eyedrops, which relieve itching and redness; and steroid and other nasal sprays, which help the nasal symptoms.

PREVENTION

There is no actual method of preventing hay fever, but precautionary measures such as those discussed above may help at least to relieve some of its discomfort.

HIVES

Hives (sometimes called nettle rash or urticaria) is a reaction of the skin marked by intense itching and, most noticeably, by the rapid development of raised smooth patches or welts (also called wheals). Hives is often a sign of an allergic reaction.

During an allergic reaction, the body overreacts to a foreign substance (called an allergen) and causes special cells called mast cells to release a powerful chemical called histamine, which is instrumental in the development of hives.

Hives is often caused by an allergy to certain foods, particularly shellfish, tomatoes, strawberries, eggs, milk, and chocolate. It can also be a reaction to drugs, food dyes, moulds, bacteria, and animal skin or hair. In addition, in a susceptible person, cold, the rays of the sun, and vigorous exercise have also been known to cause hives.

SYMPTOMS

Hives is characterised by an outbreak of red and white welts appearing suddenly either in small areas or all over the body and varying in size. They often appear and disappear, lasting anywhere from a few minutes to a day or two, but the outbreak can last for weeks. Accompanying symptoms are intense itching; occasionally, fatigue, fever, and nausea; and difficulty in breathing if the allergic reaction has led to a swelling in the respiratory tract.

DIAGNOSIS

Diagnosing the allergy and pin-pointing the allergen that is causing the trouble can require extensive testing, especially when a food may be involved. Eliminating many suspected foods, then reintroducing them one at a time, sometimes helps to diagnose the cause of hives. This must be done under professional supervision and with extreme caution. Often allergy doesn't seem to be the cause, and hives may appear for a period of time out of the blue.

TREATMENT

Hives can be treated immediately by taking antihistamines. When taken several times a day at a specific, prescribed dosage, the correct type of antihistamine will help control swelling by preventing the released histamine from triggering the hives. Drowsiness is a common side effect of some antihistamines, so the type and dosage may need to be adjusted periodically. Newer antihistamines don't cause drowsiness, but they aren't always as effective against itching. Other drug therapies such as those involving corticosteroids, which reduce inflammation, may be used to treat serious hives.

PREVENTION

Hives can be prevented by avoiding contact with the allergen or stimulus if there is one. Avoid aspirin too, as this can make things worse.

IMMUNISATION

Immunisation is the means of producing immunity, or resistance by the body to a specific disease. Doctors employ two types of immunisation: *active* and *passive*.

Active immunisation is accomplished by injecting weakened or killed viruses or bacteria into the body. This stimulates the body's natural defence system. Certain specialised white blood cells – which are manufactured in the bone marrow, are circulated in the blood, and are stored in lymph nodes and elsewhere – produce substances known as antibodies, carried in the bloodstream, that are tailor-made to fight the invading organisms. They remain in the body for years, sometimes a lifetime, to protect it against that particular disease.

Passive immunisation involves injecting ready-made antibodies – usually extracted from the blood of animals that have been immunised solely for the purpose of producing antibodies to be used in passive immunisation. Passive immunisation is borrowed immunity and is only temporary but serves to protect a person who may already be infected until the body has time to create its own antibodies.

Immunisation can provide protection against several diseases including measles, mumps, rubella (German measles), polio, whooping cough, diphtheria and tetanus.

CHILDREN'S IMMUNISATIONS

For maximum protection against diphtheria, tetanus, whooping cough (pertussis) and Hib (Haemophilus influenza B), a bacterium which is an important cause of serious and potentially fatal meningitis, a child needs a shot of the combination diphtheria-tetanus-pertussis (DTP) vaccine at two, three and four months with a separate injection against Hib, and a booster shot of diphtheria and tetanus just before entering school around age four-and-a-half. When the child gets these jabs he or she should also receive by mouth a drop of the oral polio vaccine. At 12 to 15 months a child should have a combined shot for measles, rubella and mumps.

In some areas of the country the child will be tested for tuberculosis (TB) by a skin prick at around 13 years of age, and offered vaccination if not already immune to TB.

Most GPs offer all the routine jabs, although child health clinics cover all areas too.

ADULT IMMUNISATIONS

Adults need a tetanus jab once every ten years. Otherwise, there are no routine immunisations for adults, with the possible exception of influenza shots given annually (usually in the autumn) to the aged and to patients with heart, lung, and other chronic diseases. (With the new purified vaccines, side effects are minor.) A vaccine for protection against 80 per cent of serious pneumonias is also available, to be given once every three to five years; again it would normally only be offered to elderly or chronically ill people.

There are precautions to consider. Immunisations should not be given to pregnant women, nor to anyone whose immune system is weakened by leukaemia, cancer, fever, or by prolonged X-ray or corticosteroid treatment.

INSECT BITE AND STING

Insect bites and stings are minor inconveniences to most people, but to those who have an allergy to insect venom, the consequences can be serious.

Reactions to insect venom show themselves in various symptoms: shortness of breath, rapid heartbeat, coughing, wheezing, and light-headedness. The affected area swells and becomes tender or numb. In extreme cases, anaphylactic shock (a severe reaction that can be fatal, characterised by breathing problems; hives; collapse of blood vessels; and sometimes vomiting, diarrhoea and cramps) can occur.

TREATMENT

Serious reactions to bites and stings are treated by slowing the spread of the venom throughout the body and getting emergency medical treatment as soon as possible. The venom's progress can be slowed somewhat by applying an ice pack to the affected area. Emergency medical treatment will consist of an adrenalin injection, which will weaken the reaction.

PREVENTION

Prevention of recurrent severe allergic reactions to insect venom may be accomplished with treatments of desensitisation shots; starting with an initially weak solution of insect allergen, doses are gradually increased with each shot. This allows the body to build its own tolerance to the insect venom. People with severe reactions to bites or stings should carry a syringe containing adrenalin at all times, to inject as soon as a bite or sting occurs.

Bones and Muscles

Our body's frame is an intricate structure of interconnecting parts. Every voluntary movement is the result of the coordination of the bones and muscles, as well as the tendons and ligaments.

BONES

Bones are hardened masses of living tissue that have several functions. They collect calcium for the entire body, storing 99 per cent of this mineral that is required to keep all bones firm and strong. In addition, bones produce large numbers of red and white blood cells within their softer tissue centre called marrow.

There are 206 bones in the body. Together they form the skeleton or framework for the body. The total structure maintains the body's shape and protects internal organs from injury. For example, bones in the skull shield the brain while bones in the rib cage encircle the lungs and heart.

The place where two bones meet is called a joint. This junction usually allows movement of the bones that are involved. However, movement is governed by ligaments (bands of fibrous tissue) attached to the bones and cartilage (elastic tissue) lining the ends of bones. Ligaments connect one bone with another. Cartilage cushions and protects bones with the aid of various joint fluids and bursae (small sacs containing lubricating fluid located within the joints). Other bands of connective tissue called tendons attach bones to muscles. Muscles are specific kinds of tissues that have the ability to contract. This contraction and pull on the tendon are what actually create movement of the bones. In order to move any

61

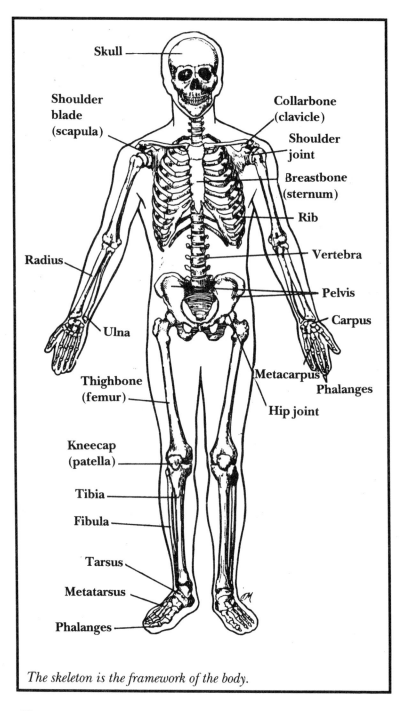

The skeleton is the framework of the body.

part of the skeletal structure, coordination of ligaments, tendons, and muscles is necessary.

MUSCLES

Body movement is effected by three different types of muscle: striated, smooth, and cardiac. Striated, or striped, muscle consists of layers of connective tissue divided into bundles of interwoven fibres running parallel to one another. These layers are attached to the skeleton, and they aid the body in voluntary movement.

Smooth, or organic, muscle lines most of the internal organs of the body, including the intestines, bladder, and blood vessels. Therefore, this type of muscle assists all functions controlled by the autonomic nervous system which governs functions under involuntary control. For example, smooth muscle helps control the flow of blood and gland secretions throughout the body, move material through the digestive tract, and regulate breathing in the lungs. Smooth muscle contains elongated spindly cells arranged parallel to one another that are often grouped into irregular size bundles. Under a microscope, this muscle appears smooth.

Cardiac muscle is the muscle of the heart, and its job is to pump blood within and from the heart. The unique characteristic of this muscle is that its fibres are striated, but they are controlled by the autonomic nervous system.

ARTHRITIS

Arthritis is an inflammation of the joints, the junction where the ends of two bones meet.

TYPES

Inflammation develops in one of two ways. With osteoarthritis, there is gradual wearing away of cartilage in the joints. Healthy cartilage is the elastic tissue that cushions the joints and prevents the bones from touching. When this cartilage deteriorates, the bones rub together causing pain and swelling. Although osteoarthritis can result from direct injury to the joint, it commonly occurs in adults over the age of 55 because of long-term wear and tear on the joints. Some people seem more prone to it because the cartilage in their joints is slightly defective, and this tendency may be passed in families.

Rheumatoid arthritis, on the other hand, can attack at any age. This form of arthritis affects all the connective tissues in the body. The precise cause of rheumatoid arthritis is unknown. Some researchers believe that a virus may trigger the disease, causing an auto-immune response whereby the body develops a sensitivity or allergy to its own tissues. However, evidence for this theory is inconclusive as yet. What is confirmed is the progression of the condition. First, the synovium, which is a thin membrane lining and lubricating the joint, becomes inflamed. The inflammation eventually destroys the cartilage. As scar tissue gradually replaces the damaged cartilage, the joint becomes misshapen and rigid.

THOSE AT RISK

Arthritis is not an inherited disease. Nonetheless, people who have arthritis in their family are more prone to develop the disease. Women have a greater tendency to develop arthritis than men, although the reason for this is unclear. In addition, excess body weight may promote osteoarthritis because of increased load on the joints. Constant joint abuse from strains of sports or employment may encourage arthritis, but inactivity can also cause the problem.

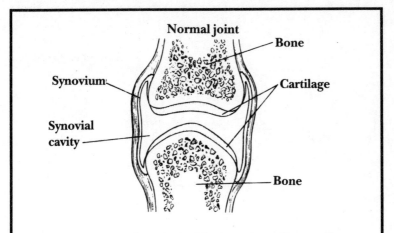

The normal joint is characterised by smooth cartilage surfaces. Synovial fluid fills the synovial cavity. There is no inflammation or debris.

SYMPTOMS

Symptoms of arthritis include swelling, tenderness, pain, stiffness, or redness in one or more joints. For many patients, pain is greater in the morning, and it subsides as the day advances. Damp weather and emotional stress do not cause arthritis, but they can make symptoms worse.

With rheumatoid arthritis, these symptoms may be accompanied by more generalised feelings of fatigue and fever. Often, this form of arthritis goes into periods of remission when symptoms disappear. When symptoms return, however, they can be more severe. If left untreated, rheumatoid arthritis may damage heart, lungs, nerves, and eyes, whereas complications of osteoarthritis can cause permanent damage and stiffness of the joints.

DIAGNOSIS

To diagnose arthritis, a doctor observes the symptoms and administers a standard physical examination. X-rays and laboratory tests may be recommended for confirmation of joint swelling.

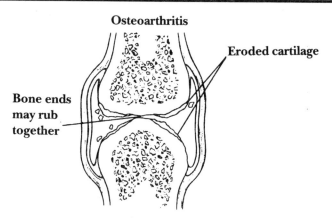

Osteoarthritis

Eroded cartilage

Bone ends may rub together

In osteoarthritis, the cushioning cartilage at the ends of bones wears away or erodes, possibly causing the bones to rub together which results in swelling and pain.

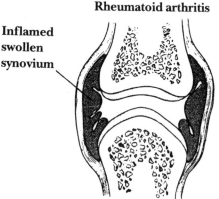

Rheumatoid arthritis

Inflamed swollen synovium

Rheumatoid arthritis is characterised by a swollen and inflamed synovium, the membrane that lines the joint and produces lubricating fluid.

TREATMENT

The most effective treatment program for arthritis consists of drug therapy, exercise and rest. Treatment should begin early after diagnosis to prevent permanent damage.

Of the drugs administered for arthritis, aspirin is one of the most useful. Doctors prescribe two to three tablets several times a day to relieve pain and reduce inflammation. To prevent stomach irritation, they suggest taking aspirin after meals or in a coated tablet form.

Often non-aspirin pain relievers and nonsteroid anti-inflammatory drugs (for example, ibuprofen, naproxen, or sulindac) may be prescribed. Corticosteroids also relieve inflammation, but they can cause adverse side effects. Sometimes, a doctor needs to try several different drugs before finding an effective one that produces no side effects.

Moderate daily exercise, such as swimming, walking, or perhaps physical therapy, is critical to maintaining mobility in arthritic joints. A supervised exercise program from a physiotherapist interspersed with rest periods helps to reduce joint inflammation. To lessen pain while increasing movement, moist heat often helps. In addition, maintaining correct posture and body weight eliminates extra burden on sore joints.

Some severe cases of rheumatoid arthritis may require surgery to remove inflamed synovial tissue. With either form of arthritis, artificial joints may be implanted to replace those damaged beyond repair.

BACKACHE

A backache is generally a gripping pain near the inward curve of the back above the base of the spine. It is one of the most common physical ailments, affecting about 80 per cent of the population at some time in their lives.

CAUSES

Pain results from a variety of causes. Strains are especially common when overworked or underexercised back muscles perform beyond their normal capacity. Muscles will then contract or go into spasm and become a tight mass of tissue. Meanwhile, the body transmits a sharp pain signal as nearby muscles tighten in an effort to protect strained muscles and prevent further damage. Strain of back muscles can be due to sports, a sudden jerking motion such as a car braking, or reflex actions like sneezing.

Overweight is a leading co-factor of backache, since excess pounds increase stress on back muscles. Similarly, pregnancy can produce back pain because of the weight or position of the unborn child. For some women, menstruation results in back discomfort.

Many people develop back pain as they age and joint tissues deteriorate or shift. Psychological tension, stress, or anxiety about everyday problems can also lead to backache. In addition, back pain can result from diseases of the kidneys, heart, lungs, intestinal tract, or reproductive organs.

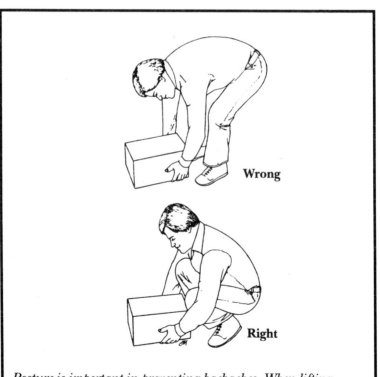

Posture is important in preventing backaches. When lifting objects, bending at the knees rather than bending from the waist keeps the weight of the object on the legs rather than on the back.

Occasionally, backache stems from a congenital (present from birth) malformation. In this case, pain usually results from unusual stresses the deformity imposes on surrounding muscular structures rather than from the abnormality itself. For example, having one leg shorter than another forces the neighbouring muscles out of alignment and may cause back pain.

SYMPTOMS

Backaches can appear abruptly after physical activity or develop slowly. The pain may feel like a sharp jab or a dull ache. Sometimes, pain becomes so piercing that a person who is bending over may not be able to straighten up. Severe back pain may also be accompanied by pain or numbness radiating down the leg(s). Most muscular back pains disappear within a week or two of their onset, while some will last one to two months, but pain may recur unless preventive measures are taken.

DIAGNOSIS

Sufferers of prolonged back pain (more than two to three weeks) should consult a doctor to check for underlying disorders such as kidney or lung problems or rare forms of arthritis, that may be causing the backache.

During the examination, the doctor asks questions about the type of pain and its location, general health, previous illnesses, and physical activity routines. The patient walks, sits, stands, and performs exercises while being observed. If an X-ray is recommended, it may or may not reveal adverse changes in the bones of the spine since not all problems can be revealed on film.

TREATMENT

If there are no physical causes for the backache, doctors usually recommend an exercise program to strengthen weak muscles. Losing weight can also relieve unnecessary pressure on the back.

For immediate symptoms, hot pads at the site of the pain will reduce soreness. Over-the-counter rubbing liniments may produce a soothing heat sensation when applied to the pain site. Doctors may also prescribe painkillers, and occasionally muscle relaxants.

When backache is the result of some deformity, surgery may be necessary to correct the problem. Sometimes, braces, corsets, or shoe lifts improve the condition. Specific exercises strengthen participating muscles and counter stress caused by the malformation. For a sudden and severe flare-up of back pain the best treatment is generally complete bed rest that allows muscles to relax and inflammation to subside.

PREVENTION

To prevent back pain, stress to the spine should be avoided. Good posture when awake and asleep relieves tension on the spinal column. Properly-fitted shoes encourage good posture, as does a semi-firm bed. Contrary to popular belief, a very hard mattress distorts alignment of the spine and causes back problems as much as a soft mattress does. You should be able to prevent this by putting a small cushion in the small of your back to support the curve of your spine as you lie flat. A semi-rigid mattress is probably best because it conforms to the arch of the back and maintains spine alignment.

Good posture is also important when performing daily activities. When lifting objects, kneeling or bending at the knees, rather than bending from the waist, keeps the weight of the object on the legs, leaving the back straight. Avoid sitting for long periods of time at a desk looking down or watching television with the chin on the chest.

FRACTURE

A fracture is a break in a bone or a cartilage, and it can be one of several different types.

TYPES

The most common fractures are the closed fracture, the comminuted fracture, the complicated fracture, the composite fracture, the greenstick fracture, the impacted fracture, and the open fracture.

- Closed fracture – one in which the skin is not broken
- Comminuted fracture – one in which the bone is broken into several pieces
- Complicated fracture – one in which significant injury has been done to internal organs, blood vessels or nerves
- Composite fracture – one in which there are multiple breaks in the bone
- Greenstick fracture – one in which only one side of the bone is broken and the bone is not severed
- Impacted fracture – one in which the ends or fragments of bone are jammed together
- Open fracture – one in which the broken end(s) of the bone pierces the skin.

THOSE AT RISK

Fractures are common among children and older people. Children have relatively soft, elastic bones. For this reason, their breaks may be incomplete, that is, they may be on only one side of the bone. Older people, particularly women, have brittle bones that tend to break easily. Hip fractures are particularly common among the elderly.

COMPLICATIONS

Among the more serious consequences of fractures are the possibility of infection and the possible damage done to the nerves, blood vessels and internal organs near the fracture.

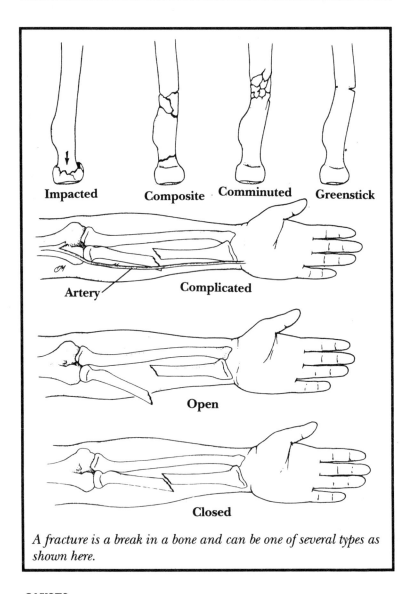

Impacted   Composite   Comminuted   Greenstick

Artery   Complicated

Open

Closed

A fracture is a break in a bone and can be one of several types as shown here.

CAUSES

Most often, fractures are caused by direct violence, such as a blow from a heavy object. They can, however, be the result of an indirect cause. A fall on a hand, for example, may result in a fractured collarbone. There are also pathological fractures, in which disease softens the bone and leads to a break.

SYMPTOMS

Among the symptoms of a fracture are pain, swelling, loss of strength, abnormal movement, and a grating sound caused when the broken pieces of bone rub together. Shock may also occur with a severe fracture if large amounts of blood are lost.

TREATMENT

Bone fractures are treated by closed (nonsurgical) or open (surgical) reduction. Reduction is a procedure in which the broken bone is manipulated, for example, by pulling or bending, so that the ends will be in the best position for healing. The pieces of bone are often held together by pins, metal plates, and rods, some of which are left in the body and others of which are removed after healing has taken place. Most fractures are treated through closed reduction. However, open reduction may be required when damage to bones, joints, ligaments, tendons or other internal parts is severe or extensive.

OSTEOPOROSIS

Osteoporosis is a common disorder characterised by a decrease in the calcium content of bone tissue that leaves the skeletal system thin and susceptible to fracture.

The chances of acquiring the disease seem to increase dramatically with age, especially for women. It seems that osteoporosis results from a loss of the female hormone oestrogen, which affects the calcium content of the bones. Menopause (cessation of menstruation or periods) often leads to osteoporosis because the body's production of oestrogen is reduced at this time. Almost one third of all women over 60 years of age have the disease to some extent.

For reasons not entirely known, white and oriental women are likelier to develop osteoporosis than black women. In addition slender females, especially those with fair skin, run a higher risk than stouter, darker-skinned women. Smoking and having a menopause at an early age increase the risk too.

Besides developing spontaneously, osteoporosis can also appear as a result of other conditions. Surgical removal of both ovaries (the female sex glands that produce oestrogen), chronic arthritis (inflammation of the joints), or Paget's disease (a disorder of unknown origin that results in bone destruction) may lead to osteoporosis. People who are inactive, either by choice or because of confinement from illness, seem more susceptible to the disorder. In addition, a diet without various nutrients, especially calcium, that promote bone development may also contribute to osteoporosis.

SYMPTOMS
Depending upon the strength of the bones, osteoporosis may initially cause either no symptoms or extreme pain, commonly in the lower back. The disease is not life-threatening, but it may lead to serious fractures which, for the elderly, can result in serious complications. Initially, sudden back pain may follow fracture of the vertebrae, the bones in the spine. This pain may lead to further inactivity which may weaken additional

vertebrae. Hence, a vicious cycle develops whereby pain leading to inactivity encourages osteoporosis which, in turn, increases bone fragility.

As the disease progresses, the spinal column may become reduced in length or may become curved due to the pressure of body weight – hence, the term 'widow's hump' or 'dowager's hump'. As osteoporosis progresses, the individual may actually lose several inches in height.

DIAGNOSIS

Often, osteoporosis progresses undetected until a fractured bone develops and an X-ray is taken. At this time, a doctor may notice that bone thinning has become a generalised condition throughout the body.

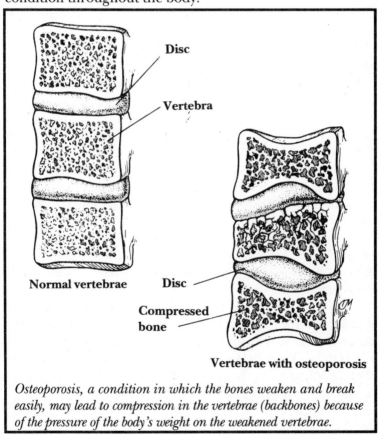

Disc

Vertebra

Normal vertebrae　**Disc**

Compressed bone

Vertebrae with osteoporosis

Osteoporosis, a condition in which the bones weaken and break easily, may lead to compression in the vertebrae (backbones) because of the pressure of the body's weight on the weakened vertebrae.

TREATMENT

Doctors urge patients with osteoporosis to follow an exercise program that will strengthen the muscles supporting weakened bones. To protect bones in the spinal column, however, lifting heavy objects should be avoided. For advanced cases, a back brace may be necessary to support body weight while sitting or standing. Crutches, walkers, or a cane may assist walking.

Sometimes, doctors prescribe the female hormone oestrogen, in the form of hormone replacement therapy (HRT) to women to decrease bone loss. Women taking these medications need careful supervision as the hormones may cause adverse side effects. Anyone receiving HRT should have a physical examination and a cervical smear (examination of cells scraped from the vagina and cervix to detect cancer) at the start of therapy. Afterwards blood pressure should be checked regularly, as occasionally it may rise on treatment with HRT.

Unless the woman receiving HRT has had a hysterectomy the doctor will give a second drug, a progestogen, with the oestrogen in order to induce regular periods. This is essential to protect against the risk of uterine cancer. Recently there have been suggestions that HRT may slightly increase the risk of breast cancer, although probably not until it has been taken for at least five years. The longer HRT is continued the better for prevention of osteoporosis, but five years seems to be the minimum time to get any benefit.

Men may be given the male hormone testosterone, which stimulates growth of body tissues, to treat osteoporosis. Recently, newer drugs have become available to treat osteoporosis in men.

For people prone to injury from osteoporosis, a balanced diet is an important factor in preventing or controlling the disease. Foods rich in vitamins and minerals, particularly calcium and Vitamin D, encourage bone formation. When the diet is deficient in these ingredients, vitamin and mineral supplements may be prescribed by a doctor.

SLIPPED DISC

A slipped disc is a back problem involving the discs of elastic cartilage tissue located between the vertebrae, the bones of the spine. The bones are loosely strung together by bands of tissue called ligaments that allow the body movement and flexibility. The function of each disc is to cushion any friction between the bones as the body moves.

When this intricate spinal structure experiences strain and over-exertion, the rim of the disc weakens and tears, rather than 'slips', causing part of the gelatinous centre of the disc to be forced out of position. In its new position, the protruding material presses against an adjacent spinal nerve and causes pain along the path of the affected nerve.

CAUSES

Most often, a slipped disc occurs when bending and straightening the back to lift heavy objects results in strain or injury. Damage to the disc may not be realised for many months, however. People with the problem frequently have a history of damage to the same area.

Discs also seem to disintegrate with age. They lose some of their fluidity and become more compressed. This form of degeneration usually results in only mild pain with intermittent backache and stiffness.

SYMPTOMS

Symptoms of slipped disc may vary with the location of the disc.

The most common slipped disc is the lowest movable disc in the small of the back. Injury to this disc causes pain along the sciatic nerve, a condition called sciatica. Mild or disabling pain and tenderness may result. Any straining, such as coughing or moving, can aggravate the discomfort. Weakness, tingling, or numbness in parts of the arms, legs, or feet may also result from damage to a particular disc.

DIAGNOSIS

To determine the source of back pain, a doctor requests a current medical history; observes the patient sitting, walking, and bending; and explores for sensitive areas by maneuvering the patient's legs in different positions, checking ankle and knee reflexes, and testing muscle strength. If needed, X-rays reveal any structural changes in bones, joints or discs.

For locating particularly problematic discs, or with a recommendation of surgery, special tests are necessary. A myelogram is an X-ray taken after dye is injected into the space surrounding the spinal cord and nerve roots. The protruding disc is detected at the point where the flow of dye is interrupted or distorted. Discography gives much the same information; but before this X-ray, dye is injected directly into the discs. Nowadays special scans such as MRI (magnetic resonance imaging) scans enable the doctor to see a picture of the disc directly.

TREATMENT

The first course of treatment for slipped disc involves complete bed rest on a firm mattress. Rest relieves pressure of the disc on the nerve and may shrink the protruding material. For moving about, some form of back support may improve comfort, but under no circumstances should a patient lift heavy objects.

For severe pain, a doctor may prescribe a pain reliever. As pain subsides, an exercise program may be recommended to gradually strengthen muscles.

Most people find partial or complete relief of slipped disc from nonsurgical therapy. However, in some cases, removing the disc surgically provides the only remedy.

Nowadays discolysis sometimes offers the same results of eliminating or reducing the disc without major surgery. With this method, the drug chymopapain is injected into the damaged disc after the patient receives local anaesthetic. This drug acts by slowly dissolving the part of the disc that is pressing on a nerve. Treatment is fast and relatively painless, but pain reduction occurs slowly, maybe in a couple weeks, if at all.

TENDONITIS

Tendonitis is an inflammation of a tendon, a band of fibrous tissue connecting muscle to bone. The condition appears most often as a result of repetitive or unaccustomed physical activity. It also can be a symptom of a more generalised inflammatory disease such as rheumatoid arthritis.

Improper activity, lack of conditioning, and poor equipment encourage the development of tendonitis. Non-athletes who suddenly begin long distance jogging or other athletic activity, or athletes who resume strenuous sports after intervals of passive activity, have an increased likelihood of the condition. In addition, people who wear shoes with rundown heels put needless tension on the Achilles tendon. Similarly, women who wear high-heeled shoes may have problems with inflamed Achilles tendons because the angle created by the shoes considerably shortens the tendons.

SYMPTOMS

A tendonitis attack causes pain in the affected tendon worsened by activity. The tendon may grow thicker than normal and be tender to the touch. Sometimes, the tendon can be very painful. When minor injuries are continually placed under stress, an already inflamed tendon could rupture and become a greater problem.

DIAGNOSIS

Doctors diagnose sports-related problems by first acquiring an exercise history to determine the patient's normal activity, and if there have been any changes in routine. A doctor also checks muscle lengths to find unusually short or inflexible muscles which may be producing the problem.

TREATMENT

Treatment for tendonitis involves resting the affected area. Pain relievers and anti-inflammatory drugs are used to ease immediate symptoms, but these preparations will not by themselves cure the condition or keep it from recurring. Injection with steroid drugs often helps and may even cure the condition. Ultrasound and other techniques from a physiotherapist may help too.

In rare cases, tendonitis patients require surgery to remove damaged tendons. Fortunately, surgical procedures have advanced in the past few years. Previously, tendons were replaced with artificial tissues that never assumed the strength and flexibility of natural tissues. Now, newer techniques and materials are being developed.

PREVENTION
People participating in sports can prevent tendonitis by taking time for warm-up prior to exercise. For example, leg and calf muscle stretching before and after running may help prevent inflammation of the Achilles tendon.

The Eye and Vision

The eye is the organ of sight. This complex structure works by capturing light and transforming it into impulses that the brain can interpret as images. These visual images give individuals information about their environment.

In order to understand visual perception, it is important to know the functions of various parts of the eye. The eye includes the eyeball (globe) and all structures within and surrounding its almost spherical mass. To guard the eye, the bony socket of the skull nestles the delicate organ. A layer of fat cushions the socket while the eyebrow, eyelashes, and eyelid provide a barrier against incoming irritants. Lining the inside of the eyelid and continuing over the exposed surface of the eyeball is the conjunctiva, a thin protective membrane. Tears (watery secretions) released from the lacrimal (tear) glands moisten the conjunctiva and keep the eyeball clean.

Light first enters the eye through the three outer layers of the eyeball. The cornea is a transparent covering over the area that admits the light. The sclera is the white of the eye (actually the tough, outer covering of the globe), and the choroid membrane contains blood vessels to nourish the eye.

Light enters the eye first through the cornea. Behind the cornea is a pigmented (coloured) structure called the iris. The iris surrounds an opening known as the pupil. The iris changes the size of the pupil depending on the amount of light present in the environment. If the surroundings are relatively dark, the pupil is enlarged to admit more light; if the environment is bright, the pupil is made smaller. Behind the iris is the lens, a transparent body held in place by elastic muscular-type tissue. The shape of the lens is changed to focus on objects at varying distances.

Between the cornea and the lens is a space, the anterior chamber, filled with a substance called aqueous humour (fluid). Aqueous fluid contains nutrients that nourish the cornea and the lens. The fluid also allows light rays to pass through the area easily.

Another chamber of the eyeball behind the lens holds vitreous humour. This clear jelly is surrounded by the retina, the innermost layer of the eyeball. In the retina are the sensitive nerve endings that convert light focused from the lens into electrical impulses. These impulses are then transmitted to the brain by the optic nerve, which extends from the rear of the eyeball to the brain.

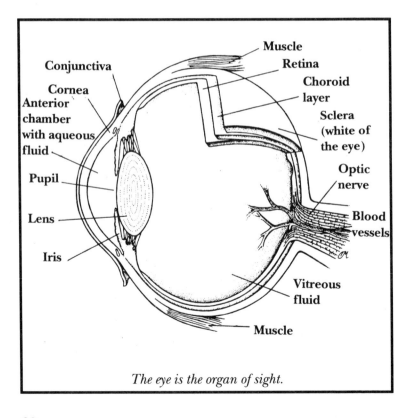

The eye is the organ of sight.

ASTIGMATISM

Astigmatism is a type of distorted vision caused by a defect in the curvature of the eye. This prevents all the rays of light entering the eye from being properly focused on the retina at the back of the eye. Some rays are misplaced, causing the image to be partially out of focus.

TYPES

Most people with astigmatism can see clearly those objects directly in front of them. However, their peripheral vision is imperfect. They may have vertical astigmatism, in which the scene above and below their direct gaze is imperfect. They may have horizontal astigmatism in which the right and left sides of their field of vision are warped; for example, a straight horizontal line may appear curved to the right and to the left. The astigmatism may also be diagonal.

TREATMENT

Fortunately, the defect in the curvature of the eye is usually uniform and can be easily corrected by spectacles or contact lenses. The fault is usually in the shape of the cornea, the clear 'window' in front of the iris and pupil, which may be slightly flattened vertically or horizontally. The spectacle or contact lenses do not bend rays entering the band of clear vision but are curved to adjust the angle of rays entering from either side or top and bottom, depending upon the prescription.

Although most people with astigmatism were born with a tendency toward the condition, a few cases are caused by eye disease or injury. These may be more difficult to correct. Regardless of the cause, astigmatism – as with any vision problem – should be corrected as early as possible. A child, in particular, with an uncorrected vision problem may develop permanently defective vision.

CATARACT

A cataract is a clouding of the lens of the eye that results in obscured vision. Because people with cataracts see their environment as if they were looking through a waterfall, the condition is called cataract from the Greek word for waterfall.

Normally, the lens is clear. Its function is to direct light into the eye so that the eye can focus on objects at various distances more distinctly. However, if the lens becomes hazy, incoming light scatters and vision blurs.

CAUSES

The exact cause of cataracts is unknown. Ageing may play a role in development of cataracts, but newborns whose mothers contracted German measles during pregnancy and some young people may also develop the condition.

Such conditions as diabetes (inability to use carbohydrates), glaucoma (increased pressure within the eyeball), or detachment of the retina (innermost layer of the eye) may lead to cataracts. In addition, injury to the lens, prolonged use of certain drugs, or high dosages of radiation (for example, prolonged exposure to X-rays) may trigger the condition.

Although usually the condition is curable, in rare cases, cataracts can cause blindness. In addition, the shadowy lens prohibits a clear view of the interior of the eye. Because of this obstruction, a doctor may not be able to detect other potentially serious eye disorders such as changes in the retina (innermost light-sensitive layer of the eyeball) or damage to the optic nerve (which transmits messages from the eye to the brain).

SYMPTOMS

The main symptom of cataracts is painless blurring of vision, occurring most often in only one eye. During initial stages of development, cataracts can cause the person to experience glare in bright light since the clouded lens scatters rather than focuses incoming light. As the condition progresses, the lens becomes milky white and vision worsens.

TREATMENT

Successful treatment involves surgical removal of the affected lens followed by the wearing of special glasses or contact lenses. With the aid of a microscope, a surgeon opens an area in the front of the eye and withdraws the lens. Local anaesthetic eyedrops make the procedure relatively painless. After a few weeks of recuperation, an eye specialist prescribes special cataract glasses or a contact lens to help correct the vision resulting from the removed lens. These aids are by no means perfect and require an adjustment period.

More recently, many doctors recommend an intraocular lens (IOL) to be implanted in the eye after the cataract lens is removed. This lightweight plastic is relatively free from distortion and closer to normal vision than spectacles or contact lenses because it occupies the exact position of the natural lens. Nevertheless, not everyone can benefit from an intraocular lens. Doctors advise patients with glaucoma, detached retina, or eye disorders caused by diabetes to wear glasses or contacts to restore vision.

Ninety-five per cent of the surgery for cataracts is without complication. Restoration or substantial improvement of vision results after surgery in the majority of the cases. When vision remains unimproved, other disorders that were undetected because of the cataract may be causing the continued problem. Generally, however, cataracts can be successfully removed and the patient can resume a normal life.

COLOUR BLINDNESS

Colour blindness is an inability to identify certain colours. By far the most common type is inherited red-green colour blindness, which affects 8 per cent of men and boys but only 0.5 per cent of women and girls. Total colour blindness, which is very rare, and pastel-shade blindness are believed to be inherited. Others, including blue-yellow blindness and red blindness, can be either inherited or acquired. Disease or injury of the retina, the light-sensitive tissue at the back of the eye, sometimes causes colour blindness.

DESCRIPTION

Colour blindness results from a defect in the cone-shaped light-sensitive cells of the fovea, the tiny yellowish pit at the rear of the eye that is the eye's centre for colour and for close work. The cone cells – seven million of them – are very different from the 130 million rod-shaped cells in the rest of the retina, which register only in black and white. The cones are believed to contain bleachable pigments for red, green and blue, colours which can combine to produce all of the colours of the spectrum. The pigments become more vivid or fade in response to colours that the eye sees. The changes of pigment produce tiny flashes of electricity that are carried by means of the optic nerve to the visual centre of the brain. There, the electrical signals are combined into a full-colour picture. In the colour-blind person, for unknown reasons, the cones are effective in other ways but the process for one or more colour pigments simply does not work right. No cure is known.

INHERITING RED-GREEN COLOUR BLINDNESS

Why is red-green colour blindness inherited by boys more often than by girls? The reason is that the defective gene for colour blindness is carried in the X chromosomes, the pair of chromosomes which determines the sex of the child. In the female, who has two X sex chromosomes, the defective gene is almost always counteracted by a normal gene in the matching sex chromosome. In the male, with an X and Y sex chromosome, there is no matching normal gene in the paired chromosome to block the defect, and the boy is born colour blind.

Red-green colour blindness cannot be passed from an affected father to his sons. Nor will his daughters be colour blind, unless the mother carries the same defective gene. However, all of his daughters are carriers of the defective gene, and his daughters' sons will have a 50 per cent chance of inheriting it and being colour blind.

CONJUNCTIVITIS

Conjunctivitis is an inflammation of the conjunctiva. The conjunctiva is a delicate membrane that lines the inner surface of the eyelid and covers the exposed surface of the eye.

CAUSES
Most cases of conjunctivitis result from disease-causing micro-organisms such as bacteria, fungi or viruses. Allergies, chemicals, dust, smoke or foreign objects that irritate the conjunctiva may also lead to conjunctivitis. Swimming may also irritate the conjunctiva – either from chlorine in the pool or from contaminated water. Occasionally, a sexually transmitted disease can cause conjunctivitis if the eyes are rubbed after touching infected genital organs.

Children contract conjunctivitis most often. Measles, a viral disease, may be accompanied by the eye inflammation. In addition, those people, both children and adults, who have allergies, such as hay fever, or who work and live in areas where they are exposed to chemicals or other irritants, are more susceptible to noninfectious conjunctivitis.

SYMPTOMS
Conjunctivitis causes redness, a grating sensation, burning, itching, and perhaps light sensitivity. Sometimes excessive

tears or a discharge containing pus occurs. Symptoms can last a few days or up to two weeks.

Usually conjunctivitis produces no permanent damage. However, if left untreated, the infection can lead to more serious eye problems. Ulcers, or eroded areas, may form on the cornea (the transparent covering across the front of the eye). Should these ulcers persist, they can scar the eye and interfere with vision.

TREATMENT

Treatment depends upon the cause and resulting symptoms of the conjunctivitis. If the inflammation is environmentally caused, simply removing the irritant may be sufficient to eliminate the condition. For more difficult cases, a doctor may prescribe antibiotic eyedrops to be used several times a day as directed. Frequent use is necessary because drops tend to be washed away by tears.

Sensitive eyes should be rested and shielded from bright lights. When the discharge glues the eyes closed, bathing them with warm boiled water and wiping with a clean cloth will loosen eyelids.

A most important fact about conjunctivitis is that its infectious form is highly contagious. Individuals with infectious conjunctivitis should not share handkerchiefs, towels or face flannels.

GLAUCOMA

Glaucoma is an eye disorder that results from increased pressure within the eyeball. The pressure builds up because fluids are unable to drain normally.

CAUSE

Although glaucoma is understood to be a problem with the eye's fluid-regulating mechanism, its precise cause is unknown. In the healthy eye, aqueous fluid in the anterior chamber of the eyeball remains under gentle pressure. When the delicate fluid balance changes, internal pressure rises in the eye. This build-up produces damage to the sensitive structures and nerve endings within the eye.

FORMS OF GLAUCOMA
Depending upon the type of defect in the fluid-regulating system, one of two primary forms of glaucoma results. Chronic, or open angle, glaucoma develops when pressure elevates gradually and normal fluid drainage slows but is not obstructed. Acute, or closed angle, glaucoma occurs when pressure mounts suddenly and forces the iris (coloured portion of the eye) into an angle joining the cornea (transparent covering across the front of the eyeball that helps focus light), thereby blocking fluid drainage from the anterior chamber of the eye.

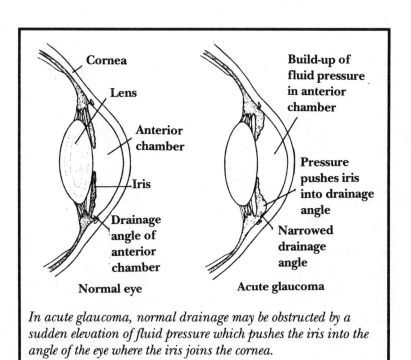

In acute glaucoma, normal drainage may be obstructed by a sudden elevation of fluid pressure which pushes the iris into the angle of the eye where the iris joins the cornea.

THOSE AT RISK

Both forms of glaucoma are more common in adults over 40 years of age. Statistics show that people with glaucoma in their families have greater risk of acquiring the condition, but inheritance has not been proven. Some evidence suggests that glaucoma may be linked to long-term use of certain drugs, especially steroids, that can alter body fluid levels. Glaucoma can also follow other eye disorders such as infections, injuries or cataracts.

SYMPTOMS

Chronic glaucoma begins with no noticeable symptoms. Vision deterioration is so gradual and painless that this form of glaucoma has been termed the 'sneak thief of sight'. Sometimes, peripheral, or side, vision loss slowly progresses as central vision remains normal. As the disorder advances, other symptoms that may be intermittent or constant include foggy or blurred vision; difficulty in adjusting to brightness and darkness; and slight pain in or around the eye, usually on one side. The one symptom indicative of chronic glaucoma is the perception of a faint white circle or halo surrounding a light. This halo is most visible in the dark while looking at a distant light.

Acute glaucoma brings sudden and severe symptoms of extreme eye pain and redness and abrupt vision blurring. Frequently, the pain can be so intense that it causes nausea and vomiting. Fortunately, acute glaucoma is rare, but when it does occur, medical attention is needed immediately to prevent permanent blindness. Usually, however, the symptoms are so severe that medical help is promptly sought.

DIAGNOSIS

If left untreated, glaucoma can lead to partial or complete vision loss. However, if diagnosed early, treatment can usually halt the problem. Because chronic glaucoma gives no warning signs, it is particularly important that people with family history of the disease be screened every year, particularly after the age of 40.

Glaucoma testing is a simple procedure. First, eyedrops anaesthetise the eyeball. Then, the doctor places a pressure gauge on the front surface of the eye to measure the amount of pressure within. In addition, the doctor inspects the interior of the eye through a special instrument that allows a view of the angle where the iris and cornea meet. This part of the examination shows whether there is blockage in the drainage system or damage to the optic nerve. Side vision is also tested by measuring the point where objects enter the patient's field of vision.

TREATMENT

Glaucoma treatment is usually effective if started early in the course of the disease. Acute glaucoma often needs surgery to quickly restore the eye's draining system. Chronic glaucoma responds well to medications. Oral drugs work by decreasing production of eye fluid, while daily applications of eyedrops promote fluid drainage. Some medications constrict the pupil of the eye to restore the drainage angle around the iris.

Other eyedrops contain beta blockers which reduce production of eye fluid without altering the size of the pupil. However, beta blockers can affect heart rate and narrow breathing passages, making these drugs unsuitable for patients with heart or lung disease.

Although chronic glaucoma responds to medication, some patients (less than 5 per cent) require surgery to open new pathways for fluid drainage. Laser therapy is the most current surgical technique. The laser (an intense light beam) generates heat, which alters tissues and cells, and stimulates better fluid drainage.

PREVENTION

The best way to prevent serious complications of glaucoma is periodic screening for early diagnosis. If glaucoma is diagnosed, attention to prescribed treatment procedures is required.

MYOPIA

Myopia, also called short sightedness, is a very common optical defect in which the eyes can see close objects clearly but faraway objects look blurred. About one in every five people is myopic; it tends to be hereditary, developing around age 12 and progressing until about age 20.

CAUSE

The defect is caused by an eyeball that is too long from front to back. Normally, the eye's cornea (the curved transparent tissue that covers the front of the eye) and lens (the disc-shaped structure just behind the front of the eye responsible for focus) refract or bend light coming from the viewed distant object so that the image focuses on the retina (a layer of light-sensitive nerve cells that line the back of the eyeball). In myopia, the focused image falls short of the retina because of the greater length of the eyeball, resulting in a fuzzy image.

TYPES

There are several kinds of myopia. Curvature myopia refers to an excess curve of the refractive surfaces of the eye causing light to enter the eye in an abnormal path. The curvature is either in the front surface of the cornea or the lens. In index myopia, there is an increase in the light-refracting properties of the lens. It is sometimes associated with future development of cataracts or iritis (inflammation of the iris). Progressive myopia is an uncommon form in which the eyeball continues to elongate, eventually leading to degeneration of the retina or a detached retina.

DIAGNOSIS

Normally myopia will be diagnosed and treated by an optician, although a sudden deterioration in eyesight should be checked by a doctor as well.

TREATMENT

Nearsightedness is easily corrected with a concave (inwardly curved) spectacle or contact lens that pushes the images back to the retina and focuses them clearly.

A surgical procedure known as radial keratotomy corrects myopia but is considered controversial. It involves cutting 16 'spokes' in the cornea coming out from the centre; as the cornea heals, it flattens and counteracts the problem. Recently, surgeons have started to use laser beams to perform keratotomy.

Myopia rarely progresses after age 30. In fact, the onset of middle age sometimes lessens the condition.

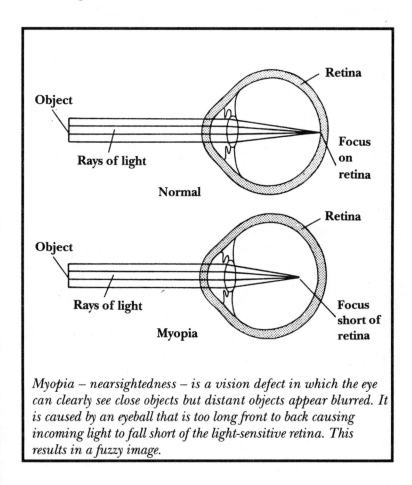

Myopia – nearsightedness – is a vision defect in which the eye can clearly see close objects but distant objects appear blurred. It is caused by an eyeball that is too long front to back causing incoming light to fall short of the light-sensitive retina. This results in a fuzzy image.

STYE

A stye is an inflamed or infected swelling of the sebaceous (oil-producing) glands in the eyelid.

CAUSES

The infection is commonly caused by staphylococcus, a type of bacteria. An external stye appears on the surface of the skin at the edge of the eyelid. An internal stye is due to inflammation, infection, or obstruction of a sebaceous gland on the inner surface of the eyelid. This type of stye is often seen as a protrusion or lump on the eyelid without visible pus or redness.

SYMPTOMS

Initially, a stye feels like a foreign object in the eye. Excessive tears, redness, swelling, and tenderness in or around a particular area of the eyelid soon follow. In addition, small, yellow bumps filled with pus may develop. These growths often burst, release the pus, and begin to heal. Once the pressure releases, the pain usually subsides.

TREATMENT

Styes generally get better on their own without treatment. Doctors sometimes use antibiotic drops or ointments, although they often aren't very effective. Warm, moist compresses applied to the eye three or four times a day may help burst the stye. In some cases, particularly in internal styes, surgical opening may be needed to cure the condition. Never should you attempt to open a stye on your own, as the risks of spreading and worsening the infection would be high.

Ear, Nose and Throat

The ear, nose and throat are interconnected, and for this reason they are often grouped together in the field of medicine. Because they are joined, infection in one structure may spread into one of the others.

EAR

The ear is the organ of hearing consisting of three parts: the external ear, middle ear, and inner ear. The pinna, or external ear, traps sound waves and directs them into the ear canal through the eardrum into the middle ear.

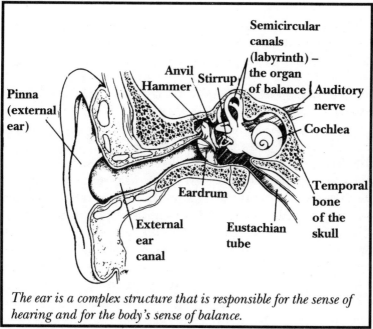

The ear is a complex structure that is responsible for the sense of hearing and for the body's sense of balance.

In the middle ear, sound waves vibrate through three tiny bones called the hammer, anvil and stirrup. Vibrations continue into the inner ear, where the cochlea transforms the sound waves into nerve impulses. These impulses then travel to the brain through the auditory nerve.

A eustachian tube in the middle ear connects the ear with the nasopharynx, the upper part of the throat opening into the nose. This tube allows air pressure in the middle ear to equalise with pressure outside the body, thus helping to prevent a ruptured eardrum. However, the eustachian tube also provides a passageway for infecting micro-organisms to enter the middle ear from the nose or throat.

Besides functioning as the organ of hearing, the ear also provides signals to the brain about the position of the body. Semicircular canals (or labyrinth) within the inner ear serve as the organ of balance by detecting motion of the head and feeding this information to the brain.

NOSE

The nose serves dual functions as the organ for the sense of smell and as an entry to the respiratory system.

When the nose works as the organ of smelling, nerve receptor cells within the nose detect smells and transmit signals to the brain through the olfactory nerve. The sense of smell also enhances the sense of taste. The ability to smell is more refined than the ability to taste; therefore, when a cold blocks nasal passages, food may seem bland and tasteless.

As an organ of breathing, the nose moisturises incoming air and filters out any foreign materials. Small glands within the lining of the nose secrete mucus, a sticky substance that lubricates the walls of the nose and throat. Mucus humidifies the incoming air and traps bacteria, dust, or other particles entering the nose. Many disease-causing bacteria are either dissolved by chemical elements in the mucus or transported to the entrance of the throat by tiny hairs called cilia. In the throat, any remaining bacteria are swallowed and killed by acids and other chemicals produced in the stomach. This efficient line of defence protects the body against the billions of bacteria continually entering the nose.

Connected to the nose are sinuses. Sinuses are cavities lined with mucus-secreting glands and filled with air, located in certain facial bones. There are four groups of sinuses – frontal, sphenoid, ethmoid, and maxillary. Their purposes are to resonate the voice and lighten the weight of the skull.

THROAT

The throat, or pharynx, is a passageway connecting the back of the mouth and nose to the oesophagus, the tube between the mouth and stomach, and to the trachea, the tube between the mouth and the lungs. Because air and food pass through the throat, the throat is considered a part of both the respiratory and the digestive systems.

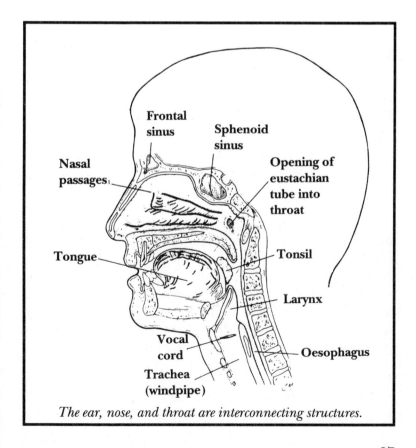

The ear, nose, and throat are interconnecting structures.

Three sections comprise the five-inch throat tube. The nasopharynx is the upper part of the throat that opens into the nose, and the oropharynx is the middle portion that opens into the mouth. The lower section of the throat, or laryngopharynx, connects the other sections with the larynx, or voice box.

Within the throat are two small tissue masses called tonsils. Tonsils help fight disease by destroying bacteria that enter the throat. This can be a formidable task, since disease can easily spread from the nose and ears to the throat.

COMMON COLD

A simple, common cold is a collection of familiar symptoms signalling an infection of the upper respiratory tract, which includes the nose, throat and sinuses.

Colds are self-limiting diseases, meaning that their symptoms last a certain length of time (or 'run their course', as is often remarked) and then disappear without leaving lasting ill effects. A cold is a mild but common disease, one contracted by adults about two to four times a year and by children six to eight times. Adults with children at home are more likely to catch colds than are those who do not live with children. Children are especially susceptible to colds because they have not yet developed immunity or resistance to the many viruses that can cause colds. Small children gradually build up immunity to viruses in their homes; then, when they go to school and have close contact with many other children, they have to combat new viruses. Similarly, adults who travel frequently or have a high number of close contacts outside their community are more likely to contract colds and to encounter new cold viruses to which they are not immune.

COMPLICATIONS
A cold can be a minor irritation, but it can increase susceptibility for more serious conditions, especially in children, the

very old, and the very weak. Pneumonia, an infection of the lungs, is probably the most serious. Ear infections, sinus infections, and bronchitis are other possible complications.

CAUSES

At least five major categories of viruses cause colds. One of these groups, the rhinoviruses, includes a minimum of 100 viruses. A different combination of symptoms and possible complications can develop from each of these viruses. It is not known exactly how viruses spread, but it seems to be a combination of physical contact and the presence of both virus particles and moisture in the air. So a virus can spread from hand-to-hand contact, for example, or from the infected person's nasal passages and throat (by droplet) into the air or onto the skin of another person. Colds have an incubation period of 48 to 72 hours, meaning that it takes that long after the virus enters the body for early symptoms to appear.

SYMPTOMS

Early symptoms of the common cold include stuffy or runny nose, sneezing, sore or scratchy throat, cough, and occasionally a mild fever. Usually, as the cold progresses, other symptoms may appear: burning or watery eyes, loss of taste or smell, pressure in the ears or sinuses, nasal voice, and tenderness around the nose.

Symptoms vary in type and severity among the various viruses, so a cold can begin with any symptom or combination of symptoms. Most colds last about a week, but about 25 percent of all colds last two weeks. Smokers and those with chronic respiratory diseases tend to display more severe symptoms, have longer-lasting colds, and develop complications more readily than do those who do not fall into these categories.

DIAGNOSIS

Since common colds are mild diseases, the doctor, in diagnosing a cold, will actually be looking for symptoms indicating a complication more serious than the common cold. Rarely, material from the patient's throat or nasal passages may need

99

to be tested for bacterial infections; a blood test may be recommended to check for mononucleosis, characterised by a long-lasting sore throat and swelling glands; or an X-ray of the sinuses may be necessary if an infection of the sinuses (called sinusitis) is suspected.

TREATMENT

Getting plenty of rest, drinking lots of fluids to prevent dehydration, and using a humidifier or vaporizer can help relieve the irritating symptoms of a cold. Nevertheless, the common cold cannot be cured, and no known treatment will actually hasten recovery. Aspirin or paracetamol are probably better than anything else to control aches, pain and fever. Many other over-the-counter medicines and preparations are available that will at least ease the discomfort. However, it is best to take specific medicine only for the symptoms actually present and to carefully follow directions on the medication package. Over-use of an otherwise effective remedy can backfire and actually make the symptoms worse, and treating symptoms that are not there can complicate matters. For example, the over-use of an antihistamine or other drying agent for nasal congestion can make a cough more uncomfortable. Or the use of a nasal decongestant for more than three days can cause more congestion, because the blood vessels in the nose which have been constricted by the decongestant tend to relax in a rebound fashion after a few days' use of a decongestant, causing even more congestion. Anyone who is pregnant or has a chronic disease should check with a doctor before using cold preparations, even seemingly harmless over-the-counter drugs.

PREVENTION

There is no known prevention for the common cold. Vitamin C has been said to help prevent colds, but many studies have shown that it has no measurable effect in this area. Avoid exposure to viruses, when possible. Boosting your immune system with regular exercise and a healthy diet, and avoiding smoking, can help too.

DEAFNESS

Deafness is a term to describe complete or partial loss of the ability to hear. There are four main types of deafness.

TYPES

Conductive deafness. This type of deafness is caused by a defect in the external or middle ear, which prevents normal transmission of sound. It may be present at birth as the result of an inherited defect, an accident in development, or an infection of the baby in the womb. It may be produced by an injury that perforates the eardrum or that breaks up the linkage of the three tiny bones – hammer, anvil, stirrup – that normally transmit sound from the eardrum through the middle ear to the inner ear. Inflammation of the middle ear, a condition known as otitis media, is another important cause of conductive deafness. Infection from an upper respiratory (breathing) tract ailment such as sore throat or flu can produce a build-up of pus in the middle ear so great that it ruptures the eardrum. Also, a plugged-up eustachian tube (the tube leading from the back of the throat to the ear) may trap fluid in the middle ear, creating temporary deafness.

Conductive deafness in the middle and later years is most often caused by otosclerosis. In this inherited condition, new spongy bone grows over the stirrup bone, preventing it from vibrating when sound travels to it through the hammer and anvil bones.

Sensorineural deafness. This type of hearing loss, known less accurately as nerve deafness, occurs because of damage to the bony structures of the inner ear, to the auditory nerve carrying sound messages to the brain, or to the hearing centre in the brain itself in the temporal lobe. It may be due to a head injury during birth, the effects of a woman's rubella infection on her unborn baby, a skull fracture affecting the inner ear or the auditory nerve, fever, bacterial or viral infections such as mumps or meningitis, tertiary (final stage) syphilis, Ménière's disease, cancers, multiple sclerosis, a haemorrhage or blood clot occurring in the inner ear, drug side effects, normal ageing, prolonged or repeated exposure to intense noise, or oedema (fluid build-up) caused by a thyroid deficiency. Most sensorineural deafness is not nerve deafness, the popular term for it. It is usually sensory deafness, caused by defects not in nerves but in the structure of the inner ear, especially in the fluid-filled cochlea and its organ of Corti which contains sensory cells that code sound waves into electrical impulses to be transmitted to the brain.

Mixed deafness. This is a combination of conductive and sensorineural deafness.

Functional deafness. This form of deafness is that which occurs without any organic defect of the hearing system or of the brain.

People with pure conductive deafness simply need louder volume to hear all sounds. Those with defects in the inner ear can hear low sounds more easily than high sounds, and some sounds may be distorted. When there is damage to the temporal lobe, the hearing centre in the brain, the person may be able to hear sounds, but has trouble recognising them and understanding words (this problem can also occur with the other types of deafness).

DIAGNOSIS

When hearing loss is suspected, a complete examination of the ear, nose and throat is necessary to identify any infections or abnormalities which might be involved. Infected adenoids or tonsils, as well as sinus or nasal infections may be linked to ear infections.

Testing for hearing loss is important for all ages, but especially for infants. Many times, partial deafness in a baby is not discovered until the child fails to learn to talk – a direct result of the hearing loss. Babies who have been born prematurely or ill, or whose mothers had certain viral infections such as rubella during pregnancy, are in special need of testing.

TREATMENT

Although at present inborn hearing defects usually cannot be corrected, deaf children can be helped to deal with their handicap. Starting very early, they may be fitted with hearing aids, may be instructed in lip-reading or sign language, and are taught to speak although they cannot hear.

Surgery to correct conductive hearing loss includes middle ear operations to replace the stirrup bone or all three tiny bones with tissue or synthetic material, to repair a punctured eardrum, and to clean out a chronic middle ear infection. Children with glue ear, a form of conductive deafness caused by fluid in the middle ear, may be helped by the placing of small tubes called grommets in the eardrum to encourage the fluid to drain or by the removal of enlarged adenoids that are blocking the eustacian tube.

A hearing aid can help to restore hearing loss in many people. It should only be purchased, however, after thorough testing of the hearing by a doctor or a specialist in audiometry, who can advise on the need for a hearing aid and on the type to buy.

PREVENTION

It is far easier to prevent deafness than to cure it. Antibiotics have made it possible to eradicate most of the middle ear infections that are one source of conductive hearing loss in children. Repeated middle ear infections may be a sign that the eustachian tube isn't working properly. Grommets, or removal of enlarged adenoids, may help. Sometimes the middle ear problems are eliminated by treating allergies that cause the eustachian tubes to close up, or by removing infected adenoids. Nerve deafness caused by continued exposure to intense industrial noise, gun shots, rock music, or aircraft engines may be avoided by wearing ear plugs or other ear protectors. Some lost hearing may return after several months of relief from intense sound. Drugs that can cause hearing loss, including some antibiotics and certain drugs that remove water from the blood, need to be used with care, and signs of hearing loss should be noted.

EAR INFECTIONS

The ear, which is responsible for both hearing and the body's sense of balance, can become infected in any one of its three parts – the inner ear, middle ear, or outer ear. However, most commonly, ear infections settle in the middle ear.

Ear infections are much more likely to affect children than adults; those most susceptible range from ages six months to six years. Children who contract ear infections in their first year are more likely to have chronic (long-term) ear infections later in life; almost every child has at least one ear infection.

INNER EAR INFECTIONS

Inner ear infections are rare, but they may result from middle ear infections and can lead to permanent ear damage. The inner ear has two parts: the labyrinth, the semicircular canals that act as the organs of balance; and the cochlea, which converts sound into nerve impulses and transports them to the brain.

OUTER EAR INFECTIONS

Outer ear infections are basically skin infections, are seldom serious, and can be treated by cleaning, with antibiotic or steroid ointments or drops. The outer ear includes the pinna (the visible ear), and the outer ear canal.

MIDDLE EAR INFECTIONS

Middle ear infections usually clear up quickly, but the more serious or persistent infections can lead to a variety of serious complications: temporary or permanent hearing loss, infection of the semicircular canals in the inner ear, facial paralysis, brain abscess, meningitis (infection of the covering of the brain), and infection of the mastoid bone, located behind the pinna. The middle ear includes the eardrum and the three tiny bones – the hammer, anvil, and stirrup – that vibrate and convey sound into the inner ear.

Middle ear infections develop when viruses or bacteria in the nose or throat travel to the ear through the eustachian tube, which connects the middle ear to the nose and throat. The middle ear also can become infected when infection spreads from a severe outer ear infection or injury.

SYMPTOMS
Middle ear infections can be recognised by severe throbbing pain in the ear; fevers up to 40° or 40.5°C (38.5° or 39°C in adults); hearing loss; and possibly dizziness, nausea, vomiting, or sore throat. Eardrums may bulge out or may even burst, oozing blood and pus into the outer ear and relieving the pain. Symptoms may worsen over hours or days. A child too young to talk may seem ill or feverish or may pull on an ear.

DIAGNOSIS
Ear infections are diagnosed by an inspection of the eardrum by the doctor. If it is red and swollen or bulging out, middle ear infection can usually be confirmed.

TREATMENT
Middle ear infections are usually quickly eliminated when they are treated with an antibiotic, often a form of penicillin. If the eardrum bursts, the outer ear must be kept clean to prevent infection from spreading.

Improved antibiotics have lessened the need for surgery, but the infected tissue, in rare cases, may need to be surgically removed. However, it should again be emphasised that this is seldom necessary because of modern, improved antibiotics.

LARYNGITIS

Laryngitis is an inflammation of the mucous membrane (or lining) of the voice box (larynx), located in the upper part of the respiratory tract. It causes hoarseness and even possibly a temporary loss of speech.

CAUSES

Laryngitis may result from a bacterial or viral infection, such as a cold or flu; from an irritation of the mucous membrane of the larynx, such as that caused by smoking; or from over-use of the voice.

Chronic or persistent laryngitis is most often caused by smoking, air pollution, dust, or smoke. It may also stem from tonsillitis, tuberculosis, early cancer, or paralysis of the vocal cords. Because laryngitis may be a symptom of a more serious condition, persons who consistently suffer from it should consult a doctor.

SYMPTOMS

Symptoms of this condition – other than hoarseness or loss of voice – include dryness and scratchiness of the throat, coughing, and pain from speaking.

TREATMENT

Laryngitis is best treated by totally resting the vocal cords. Pain may be eased with throat sprays, steam inhalations, and mild pain relievers such as aspirin or paracetamol.

NOSEBLEEDS

A nosebleed occurs when there is a break in the blood vessels in the inner lining of the nose, causing bleeding from the nose. Nosebleeds seldom require medical attention, but it is possible, although relatively rare, for nosebleeds to be symptoms of serious illnesses.

CAUSES

Nosebleeds can be caused by an injury to the nose; breathing dry air for long periods; repeated blowing or picking of the nose; tumours in the nose; or high blood pressure or other blood diseases.

TREATMENT

Very persistent or frequently occurring nosebleeds will require the attention of a doctor who may cauterise (use heat or the application of the chemical silver nitrate to seal off) the blood vessels in the back of the nose.

However, occasional nosebleeds can be treated by simply sitting up and leaning forward, so as not to swallow the blood, and pinching the entire soft portion of the nose between the thumb and forefinger for ten minutes. If the bleeding does not stop, cold packs can be applied to the bridge of the nose for 15 to 20 minutes. If bleeding still persists, a doctor should be notified.

Frequent nosebleeds from dry air may be relieved by the use of a humidifier. Also, those who have frequent nosebleeds should not blow the nose too harshly nor blow through one nostril.

When nosebleeds occur along with colds or other respiratory infections, a nasal decongestant may help to shrink the blood vessels in the nose. However, these decongestants should not be used by anyone with high blood pressure, heart disease, diabetes, or thyroid disorders, because decongestants also shrink blood vessels in parts of the body other than the nose, which can lead to complications for these patients.

SINUSITIS

Acute sinusitis is an infection of one or more of the sinuses, usually caused by bacteria and more commonly occurring in adults than in children.

In chronic sinusitis one or more sinuses are filled with fluid which doesn't drain as it should, and this may persist for months or years.

The sinuses are air-filled cavities within the facial bone structure, connected to the nose, and lined with mucous membrane. There are four major groups of sinuses: frontal, ethmoidal, sphenoidal, and maxillary sinuses.

Sinuses are normally kept clear and free when mucus drains through them into the nasal passages. If they are obstructed for any reason, such as from the congestion present during a cold, they are not able to drain properly, and infection of the sinuses can result.

COMPLICATIONS

It is rare but possible for long-lasting sinusitis to lead to more serious disorders. A persistent infection may travel to the brain or to the bone.

CAUSES

A sinus infection can be triggered by anything that prevents the mucus in the sinuses from draining properly into the nasal passages.

Congestion from colds and flu is usually to blame but other possible causes include swimming and diving, various injuries, abnormal structures in the facial bones, allergies such as hay fever, even an abscess (inflamed pocket of pus) in a tooth, which may penetrate the sinus cavities and allow bacteria to enter them.

Many different bacteria can cause sinusitis, including some of the same strains that lead to pneumonia, laryngitis, and middle ear infections.

SYMPTOMS

Acute sinusitis is characterised by pain and tenderness above the infected sinus, felt in the face, forehead, behind the eyes, in the eyes, near the upper part of the nose, even in the upper teeth (but not in a single tooth). This facial pain may be accompanied by headache, slight fever, chills, sore throat, nasal obstruction, and a pus discharge from the nose.

DIAGNOSIS

Usually a doctor will diagnose sinusitis from the description of symptoms and finding a tender area over the offending sinus. Sometimes diagnosis may include X-rays to check for fluid present or abnormalities in the sinuses and to identify exactly which sinuses are infected.

TREATMENT

Sinusitis is treated by draining the sinuses and thereby removing the bacteria that are causing the infection. Nasal decongestants, hot compresses, and dry heat all work to aid sinus drainage. An antibiotic is usually prescribed that will kill the most common bacteria that trigger sinusitis.

In severe cases, strong painkillers may be prescribed to dull the pain. Rarely, a specialist may clear the sinuses by injecting a salt water solution through the nose to flush out the bacteria.

In very rare cases, surgery may be necessary to remove a nasal polyp (a mass of swollen tissue), repair abnormal bone structures, or remove infected sinus tissue.

PREVENTION

There is some evidence that smokers are more likely to suffer from sinusitis than are nonsmokers. In addition, those who frequently have colds are more susceptible to sinusitis.

TONSILLITIS

Tonsillitis is an infection and often enlargement of the tonsils, occurring most commonly in children ages five to 15 years, and rarely in those under the age of two.

The tonsils are two small, almond-shaped lumps of tissue located in the throat at the back of the mouth. They are barely visible in infants, increase in size during the pre-school and early school years, and shrink by adulthood.

The function of the tonsils has not been exactly pin-pointed, but scientists believe that they perform at least two vital jobs: they release an antibody, or protective agent, into the throat to prevent infection from spreading into the lungs (a useful service to children, who are highly susceptible to ear, nose, and throat infections); and they attract bacterial infection and thereby stimulate the production of antibodies, which accumulate in the body in order to prevent future, and much more serious, infections. Antibodies normally do not develop unless infection is present.

If the tonsils do indeed perform these two functions, then each attack of tonsillitis may help immunise a child from disease, and once this resistance is developed, the function of the tonsils is complete.

There are two types of tonsillitis: acute tonsillitis, in which the infection flares up, then disappears in a short time; and chronic tonsillitis, in which the tonsils seem to be permanently engorged and have abscesses on them.

COMPLICATIONS
Complications resulting from tonsillitis seldom occur today, but rare cases of rheumatic fever (a disease affecting the heart valves) and infections of the sinuses, ears, or kidneys are possible.

CAUSES
Tonsillitis is caused by many different infectious agents, both viral and bacterial, the most common bacteria being streptococcus

bacteria. Acute tonsillitis is usually a virus infection. Chronic tonsillitis, however, is more of a mystery; it is not known why chronic tonsillitis occurs in certain people or what causes it.

SYMPTOMS

The symptoms of acute tonsillitis are a sore throat, fever up to about 38.5°C, chills, headache, and muscle aches. These symptoms worsen for one to three days, then subside. In addition, nausea, vomiting, stomach-ache, and swelling of glands located in the neck may also occur and may last for about a week.

The symptoms of chronic tonsillitis include a persistent or recurrent sore throat, difficulty in swallowing or breathing, and foul breath.

DIAGNOSIS

Tonsillitis is diagnosed by an examination of the tonsils, to check for redness, swelling, and a grey or yellow infectious material deposited on them. The doctor may sometimes take a sample of this material with a cotton swab in order to identify the bacteria causing the infection.

TREATMENT

Bed rest and regular aspirin or paracetamol to treat pain and fever are the most important parts of treatment. Gargling with warm salt water, or better still with a couple of soluble aspirin tablets dissolved in water, will help to relieve throat pain.

About 70 per cent of cases of sore throat and tonsillitis are caused by viruses, and won't respond to treatment with antibiotics. Antibiotics may make the remaining 30 per cent better slightly more quickly, but they don't seem to reduce the risk of other complications such as heart or kidney problems. So nowadays many doctors feel that antibiotics don't have much place in treating sore throats and tonsillitis.

Surgical removal of the tonsils (called a tonsillectomy) is seldom performed today, because research has found that even when tonsils are enlarged, they almost always shrink over time. Furthermore, removing the tonsils does not necessarily prevent recurrent sore throats or colds, as was once believed.

The Lungs and Respiratory System

The respiratory system includes the nose, the throat, the larynx, the trachea, the bronchi, and the lungs. Breathing is the process by which air flows through these structures to the lungs and by which waste gases exit from the body.

The respiratory system's function is to supply the blood with necessary oxygen and relieve the blood of the waste product carbon dioxide. This exchange of oxygen and carbon dioxide occurs in the lungs. Air from the outside enters through the nose where it is warmed, moistened, and filtered before it passes through the throat into the trachea (windpipe).

The trachea divides into two bronchi, passageways leading into each lung. Within each lung the bronchi divide and subdivide until the smallest bronchial tubes end in small cup-shaped sacs called alveoli.

It is in the alveoli that the oxygen/carbon dioxide exchange takes place. Each alveolus is served by numerous tiny blood vessels called capillaries. Oxygen in the alveolus crosses the alveolar and capillary walls to enter the blood while carbon dioxide passes from the blood through the capillary wall into the alveolus. The oxygen is then carried by the blood to the body's cells and the carbon dioxide is released by the alveolus into the outside environment on exhalation.

During inhalation and exhalation the lungs expand and contract. However, they have no muscle tissue and are expanded and contracted by the ribs and the diaphragm, the large muscle separating the chest and abdominal cavities. During inhalation the diaphragm contracts which causes it to descend and the chest cavity to expand. At this point the air pressure inside the chest cavity is less than that of the air

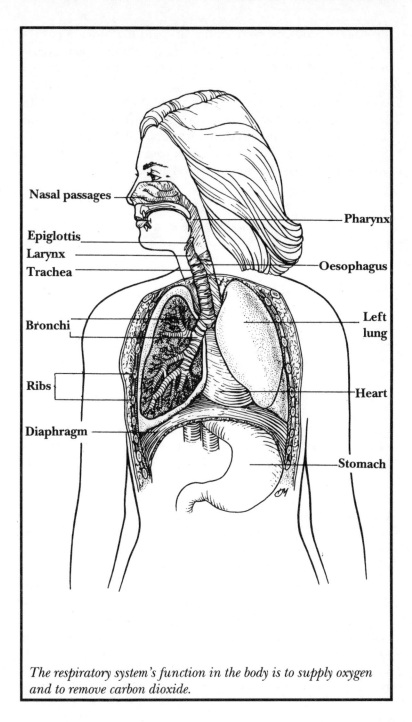

Nasal passages

Epiglottis

Larynx

Trachea

Bronchi

Ribs

Diaphragm

Pharynx

Oesophagus

Left lung

Heart

Stomach

The respiratory system's function in the body is to supply oxygen and to remove carbon dioxide.

outside the body; consequently, air from the outside rushes into the lungs. During exhalation, the diaphragm relaxes and moves up, reducing the chest capacity and pushing air out of the lungs.

The friction caused by expansion and contraction of the lungs is eased by the pleura, a thin, moist membrane that covers the lungs and lines the chest cavity. The pleura permits the surfaces of the lungs and chest cavity to slide and glide past each other as the lungs expand and contract.

ASTHMA

Asthma is a respiratory disease characterised by unpredictable periods of acute breathlessness and wheezing. Asthma attacks can last from less than an hour to a week or more and can strike frequently or only every few years. Attacks may be mild or severe and can occur sporadically, at any time, even during sleep.

The difficult breathing occurs when the small respiratory tubes (called bronchioles) constrict or become clogged with mucus, or when the membranes lining the tubes become swollen. When this happens, stale air cannot be fully exhaled but stays trapped in the lungs, and so less fresh air can be inhaled.

CAUSES

Asthma attacks can result from the bronchial system's oversensitivity to a variety of outside substances or environmental conditions. About one-half of all attacks are triggered by allergies to such substances as dust, smoke, pollen, feathers, pet hair, insects, mould spores, and a variety of foods and medications. Attacks not related to allergies can be set off by environmental conditions such as ear, nose or throat infections, strenuous exercise, breathing cold air, or even emotional stress. Heredity may play a part in the tendency to develop asthma; children with one or both asthmatic parents have a 50 per cent chance of developing the condition.

Asthma is rarely fatal, but it can be a very serious condition, especially in young children. Nevertheless, attacks often become less frequent and less severe as children grow up.

SYMPTOMS

Common symptoms of an asthma attack include tightness in the chest, difficult breathing, coughing, and the characteristic wheezing on breathing out that is caused by the effort to push the flow of air through the narrowed bronchioles. As the attack progresses, muscles surrounding the bronchioles constrict further, breathing becomes even more difficult, and mucus collects.

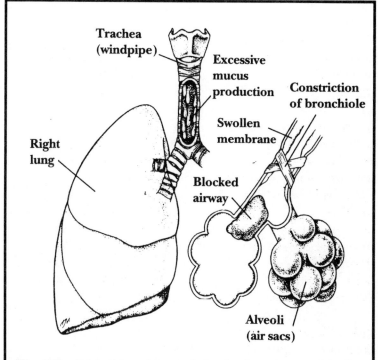

The difficult breathing characteristic of asthma occurs when the small respiratory tubes (bronchioles) constrict or become clogged with mucus, or when the membranes lining the tubes become swollen. Stale air is trapped in the air sacs and less fresh air can be inhaled.

DIAGNOSIS

Diagnostic procedures may include a complete medical history, physical examination, chest X-ray, and occasionally allergy and skin scratch tests.

TREATMENT

There is no cure for asthma, but nowadays it should be possible to keep all but the most severe cases well under control.

Drugs that relax the muscle around the narrowed bronchioles, causing them to open up, are usually taken by inhalation. This generally means breathing in from a specially designed aerosol, although modern inhaler devices which deliver a dry powder are often easier to use.

These drugs are called beta-adrenergic stimulants, and common examples are salbutamol and terbutaline. They work almost immediately and are very effective. But nowadays most doctors think that it is best to aim to prevent an asthma attack, usually by regular use of drugs that stop the inflammation and swelling of the inner lining of the bronchioles that starts an attack.

Usually these preventive drugs are inhaled too, and are either steroids such as beclomethasone or other drugs such as chromoglycate that work in a similar way. They must be used regularly, whether symptoms are present or not.

A severe attack usually responds well to high doses of steroids taken by mouth. For a short period of time these are perfectly safe, although their use over longer periods carries the risk of side effects – a risk they don't share with the inhaled steroids. Sometimes older drugs, such as theophylline, can help particularly with night-time symptoms although side effects such as nausea have made them less popular nowadays.

PREVENTION

Several precautions can be taken to reduce the possibility of an asthma condition developing. Since the tendency to develop asthma is inherited, babies of asthmatic parents should be fed breast milk or soy protein formula, since these are less likely than cow's milk to cause allergic reactions. Smoke and pet hair, as well as rugs, drapes, and overstuffed furniture, which tend to attract dust, can be removed from the home. And most important nowadays is regularly to use preventive treatment such as steroid inhalers.

One additional note: asthmatics who also suffer from angina or heart problems should take beta blocker drugs only with extreme caution, as these drugs may cause spasms in the airways.

BRONCHITIS

Bronchitis is a respiratory disease characterised by an inflammation and swelling of the main breathing tubes (called the bronchi) that connect the windpipe and lungs. When these tubes develop inflammation in their inner linings or mucous membranes, the mucous glands located in the membranes will expand and release more mucus. The bronchi, already narrowed by the swelling, become further clogged with the excess mucus. This mucus must then be coughed up in order to keep the breathing tubes free for normal air flow into the lungs.

When the excess mucus is produced and coughed up, the patient has what is known as a productive cough. A short period of productive coughing usually caused by infection is called acute bronchitis; when the coughing lingers for six months, or when it occurs for three months a year and for two years in a row, it is called chronic bronchitis. In either case, the coughing stops only when the source of inflammation has been removed or overcome and the inner linings of the bronchi have returned to normal.

COMPLICATIONS
Bronchitis alone can be fatal, but more likely it will lead to another condition that proves to be fatal. For example, in some severe long-standing cases, bronchitis-damaged lungs

can deprive the heart of adequate oxygen, resulting in death from heart failure. Also, bronchitis can be very serious when combined with other respiratory diseases. Such is the case for people who suffer from a category of respiratory conditions called chronic obstructive airways disease (COAD). Bronchitis, emphysema, and several other diseases are included in this category, and patients may suffer from two or three of the COAD conditions, or one may lead to another.

CAUSES

Bronchitis occurs when the bronchial tubes are infected or irritated. A cold, flu, or sore throat may lead to acute bronchitis, or even chronic bronchitis, if these infections occur often enough. However, chronic bronchitis is more commonly triggered by the constant irritation of environmental substances such as cigarette smoke, air pollutants or occupational dusts.

Cigarette smoking is the predominant cause of chronic bronchitis. Seventy-five per cent of all those who suffer from bronchitis are cigarette smokers. When tobacco smoke reaches the bronchial linings, it stops the action of the cilia, the hair-like projections whose job it is to sweep mucus out of the lungs, mucus that normally carries with it dust and bacteria. Once the cilia are stilled by smoke, these irritating particles remain trapped in the stagnant mucus, aggravating the delicate bronchial tubes and eventually creating a breeding ground for infection.

Some degree of bronchitis occurs in about 90 per cent of all smokers who live in polluted environments or who are exposed to occupational dusts. People who are undernourished, inadequately housed, or often fatigued are more likely to contract bronchitis. Also, this disorder tends to occur within certain families, but the reason is not yet known.

SYMPTOMS

Bronchitis can be recognised by its major symptom, the persistent cough that brings up the lung's excess mucus. Acute bronchitis may be accompanied by hoarseness, chest discomfort, slight fever, wheezing and shortness of breath as well as an increased cough. The beginnings of chronic bronchitis can be recognised by regular coughing and clearing of the throat the first thing each morning; the coughing will become more persistent and the mucus more plentiful as the disease progresses, and these symptoms may be accompanied by wheezing, shortness of breath, chest infections, and heavy panting after exercise.

As the years pass, chronic bronchitis may cause the bronchial tubes to become severely obstructed and the breathing irreversibly impaired. The heart will pump harder to get its needed oxygen and sometimes become enlarged. Nails, lips, and skin may even develop a blue tinge from lack of oxygen.

DIAGNOSIS

To diagnose bronchitis, the doctor will take a medical history, physical examination of the chest with a stethoscope, and perhaps a chest X-ray. Special machines can measure the amount of air flowing in and out of the lungs, and others can measure how well oxygen is being transported from the lungs to the bloodstream.

TREATMENT

Bronchitis is treated by removing the troublesome outside irritants, clearing the lungs of mucus, and trying to prevent infections. A chronic bronchitis patient will need to stop smoking and to avoid constant exposure to pollutants or hazardous dusts.

Humidity plays a part in treating bronchitis; patients should drink plenty of water and hot liquids, breathe warmed and humidified air from a vaporizer or humidifier, or even inhale steam from hot water or hot liquids, like chicken soup, a popular home remedy. Humid air and steam will act to loosen trapped mucus in the lungs.

A drug that relaxes the air passages, called a bronchodilator, may be prescribed to be used along with the humidity treatments.

Physiotherapy treatment may help the mucus in the chest to drain. Attacks of acute bronchitis, caused by infection, may need treatment with antibiotics.

PREVENTION

Bronchitis can best be prevented by avoiding the irritants that cause it, namely cigarette smoke, air pollutants, and dusts. Chronic bronchitis patients can prevent further irritation by maintaining good health and eating habits to avoid infections. Flu jabs and pneumonia inoculations can help to prevent infection.

EMPHYSEMA

Emphysema is a chronic, progressive lung disease. Emphysema develops when the small air passages leading to the air sacs (alveoli) in the lungs become distended and the walls dividing the sacs themselves are injured or destroyed. Spaces form where alveoli had been, and lung tissue becomes non-functional. Emphysema is commonly associated with chronic bronchitis, which is a condition in which the airways become inflamed, causing specialised cells within them to secrete a great deal of mucus. The inflammation and swelling, along with mucus plugging, result in a great deal of obstruction to air flow and cause air to become trapped.

EFFECT ON THE BODY

As the disease progresses, many complex changes take place, ultimately leading to a diminished amount of oxygen in the blood, frequently associated with an increased amount of carbon dioxide. Also, as the lung tissue deteriorates and loses its elasticity, changes also occur in the blood vessels carrying deoxygenated blood to the lungs for a fresh supply of oxygen. The net effect of all of this is that the right side of the heart, which is responsible for collecting deoxygenated blood from the veins of the body and pumping it through the lungs, must now work much harder. As the process continues, the right heart muscle is weakened by this extra work and becomes less able to pump blood into the lungs. The blood 'backs up' causing increased back pressure in the veins. This, in turn, causes the exodus of fluid into the tissues, and the result is severe swelling of the feet, ankles and legs. If this right-sided heart failure (also known as cor pulmonale) is very severe, distention of the abdomen with fluid will also occur.

CAUSES

External factors that irritate the lungs, such as tobacco smoke and air pollutants, are commonly linked to emphysema, but no one single cause has been determined. Emphysema does not stem from viruses or bacteria, as do some respiratory diseases. However, it is often aggravated by a case of bronchitis (an inflammation of the bronchial passages) or any lung infection.

In a minority of cases, emphysema may result from a genetic deficiency or an inherited lack of a blood protein that may lead to loss of elasticity in the lung's air sacs.

Those afflicted with emphysema are usually white males over the age of 50, although females are becoming equally susceptible because of increased smoking among women during recent years.

SYMPTOMS

Emphysema is characterised by one major symptom: shortness of breath. Patients may also have a persistent, racking cough, which either brings up mucus or is overly dry. Patients experience difficulty in breathing, often taking twice as many breaths as others to get enough oxygen. It has been found that advanced emphysema sufferers exert tremendous amounts of energy just to breathe. They also tire quite easily and require more calories to maintain their weight than does a normal individual. Many patients may develop an enlarged, rounded 'barrel' chest from over-inflated lungs and over-developed chest muscles used in breathing. Lips, ear lobes, skin and fingernails may become tinged blue from lack of oxygen in the blood.

DIAGNOSIS

Emphysema is usually diagnosed by several procedures, since no one single test exists to pin-point the condition. Doctors may administer breathing tests to measure the amount of air being inhaled and exhaled, but this will not reveal the disease in its early stages. A blood test may be given to determine the patient's red blood cell count; when emphysema exists with diminished oxygenation of the blood, the body will produce more red blood cells in order to carry more oxygen throughout the system, so an emphysema patient's red blood cell count may be high because of this compensation. A chest X-ray may be taken to search for specific changes in the lungs that may point to advanced stages of the disease, but a chest X-ray will not actually diagnose early emphysema. Emphysema is thus diagnosed by putting together a collection of findings.

TREATMENT
There is no known cure for emphysema, nor is it reversible. However, the progress of the disease can be checked by removing irritants, particularly cigarette smoke. Patients are encouraged to drink large amounts of fluids to help thin out the mucus that is blocking the airways. Adequate rest, a balanced diet, and moderate regular exercise are recommended. Vaporizers, humidifiers, and air conditioners help to moisturise and filter the air. Patients can learn to use their chest and abdominal muscles (with the help of a physiotherapist) to breathe more efficiently.

Several drugs may aid the emphysema patient. They act to loosen mucus secretions or to relax and expand the air passages. Antibiotics are sometimes prescribed if infection exists. In advanced cases, oxygen may need to be administered continuously. However, an emphysema patient must be particularly careful to use only the amount of oxygen prescribed. Too much oxygen can suppress the drive to breathe in some patients, thereby causing respiratory failure and possibly death. In addition, sedatives and sleeping medications should be avoided by patients with severe emphysema as these can also lead to a dangerous slowing of breathing.

Emphysema is a very serious condition. However, with the help of modern treatments, breathing aids, and medications, most patients can lead a reasonably comfortable life. It is, however, necessary for these individuals to stop smoking and avoid air pollutants as much as possible.

PNEUMONIA

Pneumonia is an infection of the lungs in which tiny air sacs in one or more sections of the lungs become inflamed and filled with fluid and white blood cells, which try to fight off the infection. It can be fatal, usually for the very young and very old.

TYPES

There are several types of pneumonia, distinguished by the part of the lung that is infected. Lobar pneumonia is an infection in only one section, or lobe, of the lungs. Double pneumonia is an infection in a lobe or lobes of both lungs. Bronchopneumonia, a complication of acute bronchitis, is the term used to describe an infection in the section of the lungs near the bronchi (the airways connecting the windpipe and lungs).

Pneumonia most often strikes the person whose resistance is lowered, often by another upper respiratory tract infection or a systemic (bodywide) disease. It is often a secondary disease stemming from inadequate defence mechanisms, from cold or flu, or from long-term diseases, such as chronic bronchitis, emphysema, asthma, diabetes, cancer, or sickle-cell anaemia.

CAUSES

Viruses, bacteria, and occasionally fungi or other micro-organisms may cause pneumonia. Also, it may develop if a person inhales certain chemicals or if food, vomit or a foreign object passes through the trachea (the windpipe) instead of the oesophagus (the passageway from the mouth to the stomach) and settles in a lung. Smoking, excessive drinking, a prolonged period in bed, anaesthesia, sedatives, and immune-suppressing drugs may make an individual more likely to develop pneumonia if exposed to an infectious organism. Pneumonia is most common during flu and cold epidemics and during the winter months when people are indoors where bacteria and viruses are easily spread.

123

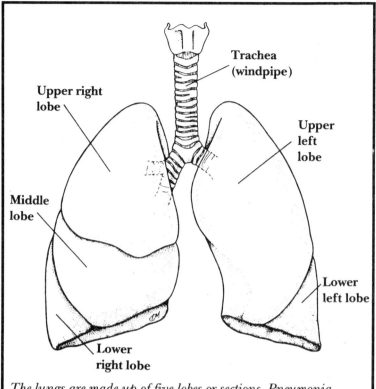

The lungs are made up of five lobes or sections. Pneumonia affecting one lobe is called lobar pneumonia. If pneumonia strikes a lobe or lobes in both lungs, it is called double pneumonia.

SYMPTOMS

All types of pneumonia are characterised by four major symptoms: chest pain, a sudden rise in temperature, coughing, and difficult breathing. Viral pneumonia, more common and generally less serious than other varieties, is recognised by coughing and other cold symptoms, as well as by general fatigue. Also, fever, chest pain, and difficult breathing may signal the presence of this disorder. Bacterial pneumonia generally comes on suddenly with shaking chills and a rapid, steep rise in temperature; shallow breathing; and a cough that brings up a bloody, dark yellow or rust-coloured sputum. An oxygen shortage that sometimes accompanies bacterial pneumonia will be indicated by other symptoms such as headache; nausea; vomiting; and cyanosis, a blue discoloration of the lips and fingertips.

DIAGNOSIS AND TREATMENT
Pneumonia is diagnosed by listening to the chest with a stethoscope in order to detect the presence of fluid in the lungs; X-rays and an analysis of the discharge that is coughed up may also help to identify pneumonia.

Viral pneumonia is usually treated with commonsense remedies: staying in bed; drinking lots of fluids; maintaining a light diet; and using pain relievers to combat discomfort.

The more serious bacterial pneumonia, however, requires antibiotics such as penicillin. Patients also need to stay in bed, or, if the case is serious enough, enter hospital for care and supervision. If breathing difficulty worsens, oxygen may be administered.

PREVENTION
There are vaccines that may help in preventing some types of pneumonia. Pneumonia caused by pneumococcus, the most common bacterial cause of pneumonia, can be prevented with a vaccine and it is especially recommended for the elderly or for those with chronic diseases that may weaken the respiratory system. Viral pneumonia caused by certain flu viruses may be prevented with a vaccination against influenza A, a virus which often leads to pneumonia.

The very young, the very old, and the chronically ill are the most likely to contract pneumonia, so care must be taken to protect those who fall into these categories from respiratory infections.

The Heart and Circulatory System

The circulatory system, which includes the heart, the blood vessels and the blood, nourishes every part of the body.

HEART

The heart is a hollow, muscular organ that is the basis of the circulatory system, which maintains blood circulation throughout the body. The organ lies behind the sternum, or breastbone, between the lungs; and its size in most adults approximates that of a clenched fist. A normal heart can beat from 60 to 90 times per minute. A heartbeat is the rhythmic contraction of heart muscle pumping blood.

Blood passes through four chambers in the heart separated by valves. Valves control movement of blood among these compartments. First, blood flows from the veins into the right atrium or upper right chamber. The fluid continues down to the right lower compartment, or right ventricle. From this chamber, the blood is pumped into the lungs to exchange carbon dioxide (waste product from cells) for oxygen (element necessary for cell life). This rejuvenated blood then returns to the heart into the upper left chamber, or left atrium, which pumps the blood down into the lower left chamber, or left ventricle. From here, the left ventricle forces blood away from the heart through the aorta (main artery or passageway that extends through the chest and abdomen) to arteries that carry the blood to all the tissues of the body.

BLOOD VESSELS

Blood vessels comprise the network of passageways transporting blood throughout the body. This complex system consists

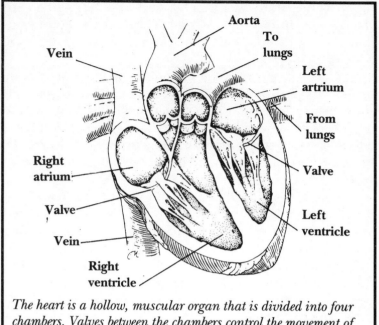

The heart is a hollow, muscular organ that is divided into four chambers. Valves between the chambers control the movement of blood between the chambers. The heart acts as a pump to maintain the circulation of blood.

of various types of blood vessels that are defined according to their size, function, and physical properties. Arteries can be large and elastic, medium-sized and muscular, or small (called arterioles). Their job is to receive blood from the heart and move it out to body tissues.

In the tissues, smaller sub-divided arteries, called capillaries, exchange nutrients for waste products. Then, veins carry the 'used' blood back to the heart to be recirculated through the lungs and then back through the heart and arteries to the body.

BLOOD
Blood is the fluid that travels in blood vessels throughout the body transporting oxygen and other nutrients to the tissues and carrying waste products away from the tissues. It consists of plasma, a faint yellow liquid comprised of protein and water. Within the plasma are three formed elements – red

127

blood cells, white blood cells, and platelets – that are visible only under a microscope. These elements are manufactured by the soft tissue, called bone marrow, in the centre of bones.

Red blood cells carry oxygen from the lungs to various body tissues. Oxygen travels attached to haemoglobin, a pigmented substance in red blood cells that contains iron. When the amount of haemoglobin or the total number of red blood cells falls below a specified amount, anaemia develops. Normally, there are about 27 million red blood cells in one teaspoon of blood.

The job of the white blood cells is to protect the body from invading organisms. Whenever the body becomes wounded or infected, white blood cells attack and kill disease-causing agents in the affected area. In addition, certain white blood cells produce antibodies. These substances counteract harmful agents by destroying or inactivating them so they are powerless. Because the body produces more white blood cells in response to infection, any change in their number signals disease. From 25 000 to 50 000 white blood cells exist in one teaspoon of blood.

Platelets are small colourless discs numbering between 750 000 to 1 750 000 in a single teaspoon of blood. They work to help the blood clot.

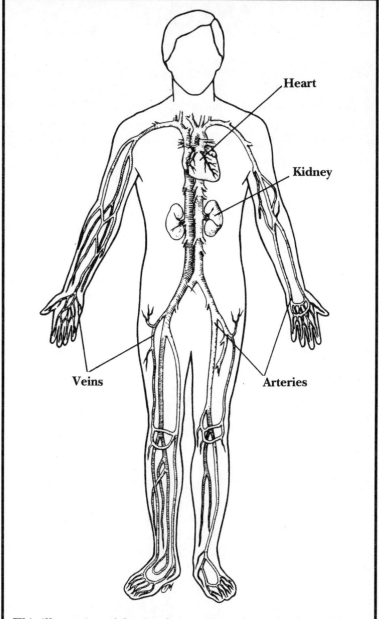

This illustration of the circulatory system shows the heart, the kidneys, and the major arteries (left side of the body) and major veins (right side of the body).

ANAEMIA

Anaemia is a general term referring to a shortage of red blood cells or a reduction of their haemoglobin content. Haemoglobin is the pigment (coloured agent) in the blood that carries oxygen in the blood cells. Therefore, a shortage of red blood cells or haemoglobin means that the blood will be unable to carry adequate oxygen to all parts of the body.

TYPES
There are many types of anaemia, such as iron deficiency anaemia, folic acid deficiency anaemia, pernicious anaemia (Vitamin B_{12} deficiency), aplastic anaemia, and various haemolytic anaemias (in which red blood cells are broken up) including sickle-cell anaemia. Each type has its own cause and therefore its own methods of treatment, but all types of anaemia are the result of an excessive loss or destruction of red blood cells or an inadequate production of red blood cells and haemoglobin.

CAUSES
Anaemia can be caused by vitamin deficiencies or the body's inability to absorb certain vitamins, the destruction of red blood cells, inherited abnormalities in the blood, or the bone marrow's failure to manufacture red blood cells. Such diverse conditions as bleeding ulcers, drug allergies, cancer, and exposure to radioactivity, can lead to anaemia.

People with poor diets or histories of alcoholism are more likely to develop one of the anaemias caused by vitamin deficiencies. Women are particularly susceptible to iron deficiency anaemia (a shortage of the mineral iron, which is necessary to produce haemoglobin) because of regular loss of blood during menstruation as well as depletion of iron during pregnancy by the unborn baby. A tendency toward anaemia can also be inherited, in the form of sickle-cell anaemia, for instance.

Anaemia can range from a severe case which may lead to

extreme exhaustion or even death, to a mild condition which may be recognised only by a persistent tiredness.

SYMPTOMS
The symptoms of anaemia are fatigue, shortness of breath, pounding and increased heartbeat, headaches, loss of appetite, dizziness, ringing in the ears, and weakness or faintness. Burning of the tongue, and/or a change in its appearance, may also be a clue. A physical sign of anaemia may be paleness in the creases of the palms, under the fingernails, and in the lining of the eye. Very severe cases may be signalled by swollen ankles and other signs of heart failure, and shock.

DIAGNOSIS
Diagnosis includes a physical examination as well as tests of the blood and often the bone marrow to detect shortages of red blood cells or haemoglobin.

TREATMENT
Each type of anaemia has different causes and therefore different treatments. *Iron deficiency anaemia* is caused by a shortage of the mineral, iron, which is necessary to produce haemoglobin. This shortage can be caused by a variety of conditions: a drastic blood loss, such as from an accident, or a chronic blood loss, such as from a bleeding ulcer or excessive menstrual flow; hookworm; a diet lacking in dark green vegetables and meat, which are good sources of iron; and pregnancy. This type of anaemia can be treated with iron supplements (for example ferrous sulphate or ferrous gluconate tablets).

Folic acid deficiency anaemia is caused by insufficient folic acid in the diet, also necessary for haemoglobin production. This deficiency may be caused or aggravated by malnourishment and alcoholism. Some disorders of the small intestine, such as inflammatory bowel disease, may also cause it. It is treated with folic acid and sometimes additional vitamin supplements.

Pernicious anaemia is caused by the body's inability to absorb Vitamin B_{12}, necessary for the production of red blood cells in the bone marrow. A substance called the intrinsic factor, which helps to absorb Vitamin B12, is lacking in the stomach of someone suffering from this condition. Pernicious anaemia is treated with Vitamin B12 injections directly into the bloodstream, bypassing the stomach completely. Inability to absorb Vitamin B12 can be caused by some parasites, inflammatory bowel disease, and other diseases of the small intestine.

Aplastic anaemia is caused by the bone marrow's inability to produce blood cells. This deficiency affects the production of white and red blood cells, as well as the platelets (the blood cells that work to coagulate or clot the blood). The bone marrow's ability can be inhibited by cancer or exposure to radioactivity, hazardous chemicals, or some drugs. This variety of anaemia is treated with blood transfusions and bone marrow transplants. It is a serious condition.

Haemolytic anaemias are caused by the destruction of red blood cells. These anaemias can be either acquired (developed over time) or congenital (present at birth).

Acquired haemolytic anaemias can be caused by mismatched blood transfusions, a drug allergy, cancer, or a serious infection. Treatment of the source is necessary to treat the resulting anaemia; blood transfusions can treat the condition temporarily.

Congenital haemolytic anaemias are caused by an inherited abnormality in the red blood cells. The most common type is *sickle-cell anaemia*, a disorder that strikes mostly black people, in which the red blood cells, sickle-shaped instead of disc-like, cannot carry enough oxygen throughout the body. These cells are also very fragile and break easily (or haemolise). This disease is characterised by crisis period bouts of severe joint or abdominal pain and can lead to complications such as kidney disease, gall-stones and heart failure. Sickle-cell anaemia is treated with painkillers, oxygen, and transfusions. Avoiding situations in which oxygen may be scarce, such as high altitudes, is advisable.

PREVENTION

There are no specific methods to prevent anaemias other than a balanced diet to prevent anaemia caused by vitamin and mineral deficiencies.

ANEURYSM

An aneurysm is a bulge in a blood vessel, usually an artery, due to a weakness in the vessel wall particularly in the elastic, muscular layer of the artery wall. An artery has three layers: the intima, which is the smooth inner layer; the media, composed of the elastic and muscular fibres; and the adventitia, the tough outer layer. A true aneurysm involves all three layers, whereas a 'false' aneurysm is a disruption and/or clot in one or two of the layers causing a bulge in the vessel. A dissecting aneurysm occurs when blood enters the layers of the media, causing it to become separated from the other layers, thereby creating an extra channel through which blood flows and is diverted from the organs. This dangerous condition can develop rapidly, in hours or days. Once between the media layers, the blood keeps creating a new channel that may finally extend the full length of the artery.

The main danger of most untreated aneurysms is that they may rupture or dissect causing death from loss of blood. If death does not occur, blood loss may so decrease blood flow to the heart that the heart cannot work properly.

CAUSES

There are various causes of aneurysms. Those occurring in the arteries of the brain are often due to a genetic (inherited) defect – a weakness in or lack of elastic tissue in the media. If they rupture, a stroke can result.

Aneurysms in the small arteries may be caused by blood infections that weaken the vessel wall. Penetrating wounds occasionally can cause aneurysms. The sexually transmitted disease syphilis may also be a cause of aneurysms. Syphilis can cause an inflammation of the microscopic arteries that feed a large one (this is called vasculitis). When this occurs, these small arteries are lost, thereby causing a loss of nourishment to, and a dying off and scarring of, parts of the large arterial wall. This process leads to weakness of the wall and consequent formation of an aneurysm.

Dissecting aneurysms usually occur in the aorta (the main blood vessel leading away from the heart through the chest and abdomen), with atherosclerosis (hardening and scarring of the arteries) the most common cause, especially in the elderly. However, when dissecting aneurysms occur in the young, the cause is usually an inherited condition that results in damage to the media.

SYMPTOMS

Symptoms of dissecting aneurysms of the aorta, if in the chest, include sudden, severe pain in the area of the aneurysm, often resembling a heart attack. There may be pain under the breastbone or in the back of the neck, difficulty in swallowing, shortness of breath, hoarseness, or a heavy cough. An aneurysm in a neck artery may create a pulsating swishing sound that the patient can detect.

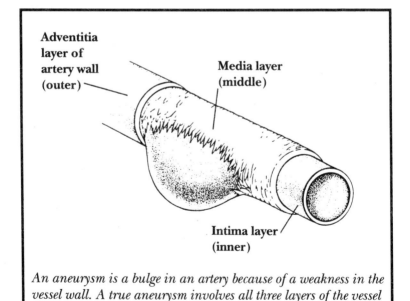

An aneurysm is a bulge in an artery because of a weakness in the vessel wall. A true aneurysm involves all three layers of the vessel wall, whereas a 'false' aneurysm, shown here, is a disruption in one or two of the layers causing a bulge in the vessel.

Evidence of an aneurysm can be a tender, pulsating mass in the abdomen, or a painful, tender mass at the back of the knee (the latter can lead to blood clots that can travel downward and may result in death of tissue and gangrene in the toes). Symptoms of dissection or rupture in the abdomen can include sudden, severe central or low abdominal pain radiating to the back; a loss of blood flow to the legs; and shock – collapse of circulation with fainting, pale and clammy skin, and rapid weak pulse. Death can result quickly.

DIAGNOSIS

X-ray and ultrasound pictures are taken of affected areas and used to locate aneurysms and determine their extent. The most reliable test is called an arteriogram or angiogram. In this test an X-ray dye is injected directly into the aorta providing an excellent visual picture on an X-ray.

TREATMENT

Treatment of most aneurysms, especially dissecting aneurysms, should begin as soon as possible. Patients with dissecting aneurysms belong in an intensive care unit. Drugs are given to lower high blood pressure (which worsens a dissecting aneurysm) and thus to reduce the chances of rupture. Occasionally, under lessened pressure, a dissecting aneurysm heals itself. Long-term medication which keeps blood pressure low is one possible treatment for those who cannot be operated on. Surgery, however, is by far the most satisfactory solution where it is possible. The damaged portion of the blood vessel is removed and replaced with a synthetic or natural vessel. Patients with ruptured aortic and, in most cases, dissecting aneurysms need emergency surgery. Rapid replacement of blood is necessary, as is intensive monitoring. Surgery for aneurysm is usually long and difficult. However, with newer methods of diagnosis, many more people are being spared the risks of surgery by correction of the aneurysm before it becomes a problem.

ANGINA PECTORIS

Angina pectoris, usually referred to simply as angina, is a warning signal in the form of chest pain, commonly dull and pressure-like, indicating that the heart muscle is getting insufficient blood and therefore insufficient oxygen. Angina occurs when the heart is using oxygen beyond what its blood supply can provide and is a sign that the body needs to slow down to permit the heart to catch up.

An angina attack is not a heart attack. Its pain is usually not as severe or as long-lasting as that experienced during a heart attack, and it does not destroy the heart muscle, as does a heart attack. However, those who suffer from this condition have a greater risk of a heart attack than those who do not.

CAUSES

Angina can be caused by any number of factors that prevent the heart muscle from getting enough blood from the circulatory system. By far the most common cause of angina is coronary artery narrowing due to atherosclerosis. The coronary arteries supply the heart muscle itself with blood. When an increased demand is placed upon the heart by the body, for instance by exercise, the heart must work harder to supply blood (and thereby oxygen) to keep the muscles and organs nourished. This increased work effort causes the heart muscle itself to require more blood. When narrowing of the coronary artery is present, the areas of heart muscle supplied by that part of the coronary artery cannot get enough blood in time to keep up with the demand. When this occurs, the muscle reacts by causing pain – angina pain. Exercise, stress, or even cold weather can trigger an attack.

This pain usually occurs during or after physical exertion or emotional stress, lasts only three to five minutes, and is relieved by resting or relaxing. If the pain does not go away within five minutes or if the pain increases in severity, the condition causing it may not be angina. It may be another disorder unrelated to the heart or it may be a heart attack.

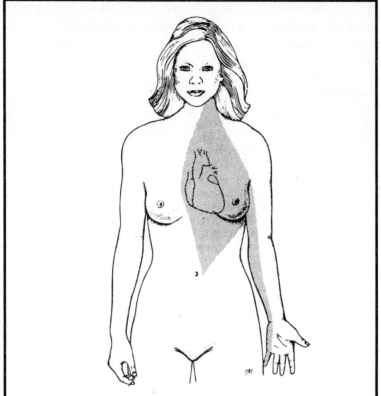

Although anginal pain is most often felt in the chest, it can also be felt below the breastbone near the uppermost part of the abdomen and along the neck. Pain and numbness may also extend down the arm and wrist to the little finger especially on the left.

Overeating and smoking can also trigger and aggravate angina; overeating by drawing much-needed blood to a full stomach to aid in digestion, and smoking by causing the coronary arteries to contract thus reducing the oxygen-carrying capacity of the arteries.

RISK FACTORS

Several so-called 'risk factors' are associated with the development of coronary artery disease and angina. Family history of heart attack, smoking, high cholesterol levels, and possibly high blood pressure, are among the best-known. There is much controversy in medicine regarding the degree of impact these factors have. However, there is much evidence favouring reduction of any and all of these factors. Furthermore, common sense would dictate that one attempt to do this.

SYMPTOMS

The major symptom of angina is a dull pressure or a sensation of squeezing in the centre of the chest behind the breastbone. This dull pain in the chest is often compared to that accompanying indigestion. Angina pain can also be felt in the uppermost part of the abdomen and along the neck, and numbness may extend down the arm and wrist to the little finger, especially on the left. The bodily location and severity of the pain vary among angina patients, but the same symptoms usually reoccur for the same patient with each incident.

DIAGNOSIS

Angina is diagnosed by first eliminating the possibility that the pain is originating from some other disorder, such as gallbladder disease, rib injury, muscle spasm, or pleurisy (an inflammation of the membrane that covers the lung). The doctor will take a complete medical history, physical examination, and probably an exercise or stress test using an ECG (electrocardiograph) which measures the heart's electrical impulses during exercise. This test can indicate abnormalities in the arteries that are preventing sufficient blood to flow to the heart. Also, radio-active isotopes or X-ray opaque fluids can be injected into the bloodstream to monitor the flow of blood through the heart. The most definitive tests for the diagnosis of coronary artery disease are cardiac catheterisation and angiogram. In the angiogram, a radio-opaque (able to be seen on X-rays) dye is injected through a tube (catheter) placed directly into the heart through an artery in the leg or arm. Once the dye is injected, X-ray films are taken, and the areas of obstruction to the dye within the coronary arteries can be clearly seen. During cardiac catheterisation, other important information, such as the overall condition of the heart muscle, can also be obtained.

TREATMENT

Angina is often treated by recommending changes in the patient's lifestyle, to reduce the strain on the heart, and by administering medication, to modify the supply-demand relationship of the heart muscle and its blood supply.

A change in lifestyle will be necessary for patients who smoke, overeat, or overexert themselves. Certain types of violent exercise may be too stressful, but regular exercise is necessary to improve collateral circulation (the natural development of a system of small blood vessels that detour obstructions in the arteries and supply blood directly to the heart).

The medication most often used to treat angina attacks is nitroglycerin, which may act by expanding blood vessels to increase blood flow and/or by altering the distribution and volume of blood in the heart. Nitroglycerin is taken in the form of a tablet that is dissolved under the tongue, or a mouth spray. Pain should stop within three or four minutes; if it does not, the pain may not be due to simple angina. Nitroglycerin can also be prescribed as a skin patch. This is used for the prevention of attacks, not for the treatment of an acute episode.

Surgery to bypass the obstructions in the arteries is performed only when angina cannot be controlled with medication or when its pain is becoming increasingly severe. There has been much controversy surrounding bypass surgery, mainly centring around the question of whether this procedure can increase life expectancy in those with coronary artery disease and angina. At present, there is no question that the surgery relieves pain and allows for greater exercise tolerance in the majority of patients who undergo it for severe angina. In certain patterns of disease such as obstruction of the 'left-main' coronary artery, the operation definitely prolongs life expectancy. In other patterns such as 'triple vessel disease' where branches of all three coronaries (except for the left-main) are involved, the surgery most likely allows a longer life. In still other patterns, the question is unsettled. Whether or not the surgery will prevent a heart attack is also an unsettled issue.

PREVENTION
Incidents of angina pain can be prevented with several drugs: nitrates and calcium antagonists (drugs such as nifedipine and verapamil that act by blocking the constricting actions of calcium on arterial muscle), which have a longer lasting effect than plain nitroglycerin and may be taken on a regular basis; and beta blockers, which also effectively prevent angina, since they decrease the work of the heart, thereby lessening its oxygen needs and making it less likely that angina will occur. (One additional note: beta blockers should be used with caution if at all by asthma patients, as these drugs may cause spasms in the breathing tubes and subsequent breathing difficulties.)

ATHEROSCLEROSIS

Atherosclerosis is a slow, progressive disease of the arteries in which various fatty deposits partially clog or, eventually, totally block the blood flow. It is often called 'hardening of the arteries'.

COMPLICATIONS
This blockage of various arteries can result in serious complications when the arteries involved lead to vital organs: heart attack can result when an artery to the heart is totally blocked, and angina pectoris (chest pain) can be caused by partial clogging of an artery; stroke occurs when an artery to the brain is blocked; kidney disease can develop from obstruction in the arteries leading to the kidneys; blindness or diseases of the extremities can result from blockages of the arteries supplying these areas of the body.

DESCRIPTIONS
Atherosclerosis occurs when the normally smooth, firm linings of the arteries have become roughened, thickened, and clogged with deposits of fat, fibrin (a clotting substance),

calcium, and cellular debris. This condition develops over time, in a step-by-step procedure. Fats (called lipids), necessary for the production of certain hormones and tissues, are constantly present in the bloodstream. When the level of these fats is greatly increased, however, fatty streaks form along the artery walls. These streaks, harmless in themselves, can cause small nodules of fatty deposits (cholesterol) to jut out from the normally smooth linings of the artery walls. Fibrous scar tissue grows under these nodules and further attracts calcium deposits; accumulated calcium develops into a hard, chalky film called plaque that cannot be removed. This permanent coating inside the arteries hampers their ability to expand and contract properly and slows the blood flow through the now narrowed channels. Clots may now easily form, totally preventing the blood from travelling through the artery.

CAUSES

The exact cause of this process has not been pin-pointed, but the initial increase of the blood's fat content may be triggered by diets high in saturated fats (fats that are usually solid at room temperature, including all animal fats such as those found in butter and meats). Also, the body's inability to absorb these fats from the bloodstream may lead to their increased build-up in the arteries.

Hypertension (high blood pressure) can increase the risk of atherosclerosis because it puts constant strain on the arteries, thus speeding up the clogging and hardening process. Smoking narrows the arteries, thus restricting blood flow and inviting atherosclerosis to set in.

SYMPTOMS

Atherosclerosis alone has no visible symptoms. In fact, the disease often remains undetected until the arteries are totally blocked, and strain or damage to the affected organs produces symptoms. For example, if an artery supplying the heart is afflicted with atherosclerosis, chest pain may be felt; if atherosclerosis affects a head artery, the patient may experience dizziness, blurred vision, and faintness.

141

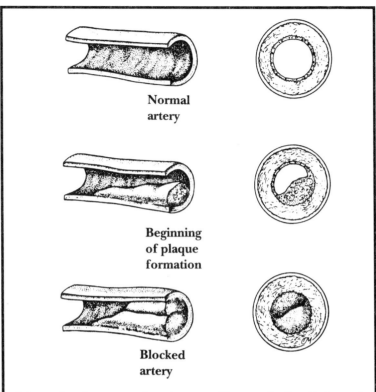

**Normal
artery**

**Beginning
of plaque
formation**

**Blocked
artery**

*Atherosclerosis occurs when the normally smooth, firm linings of
the arteries become roughened and thickened with deposits of fat,
calcium, and cellular debris. Developing into a hard film called
plaque, this deposit eventually may build up and block the artery.*

DIAGNOSIS

Diagnosis of atherosclerosis involves several methods: an
exercise tolerance or stress test using an ECG (electrocardiograph), which measures the electrical impulses generated by
the heart and which will indicate damaged heart tissue or
blocked arteries; ultrasound, which records blockage in the
arteries, abnormalities of the heart chambers and valves, and
the movement of blood through the heart; and radioactive
isotopes or X-ray opaque fluid, which, when injected into the
bloodstream, can be traced through the circulatory system to
indicate obstructions or areas insufficiently supplied with blood.

TREATMENT

Treatment of this disorder aims at reducing the strain on the heart and preventing further artery damage. Changes in lifestyle and eating habits along with the administration of medication can accomplish this. Currently there are no available medications that will actually dissolve the deposits that have clogged the arteries. Delicate surgical procedures, however, may be performed to remove those deposits that are blocking arteries to vital organs. These procedures, called endarterectomies, are performed on relatively large vessels such as those entering the brain, heart, kidneys, and legs. Surgery cannot remove deposits in small blood vessels of these organs.

Lifestyle changes include cutting out smoking; reducing cholesterol intake; perhaps losing weight (obesity puts a strain on the heart); and maintaining a moderate, but not overly strenuous, exercise program (exercise helps develop the collateral circulation, a system of small blood vessels that can bypass the partially blocked arteries and directly supply organs with blood).

Several drugs have been developed to try to increase blood flow through atherosclerotic vessels, but unfortunately they don't often offer much relief. If atherosclerosis has led to angina, several other drugs may help to suppress chest pain by expanding the arteries and increasing blood flow; they are nitroglycerin, nitrates, and calcium antagonists. If high blood pressure contributes to the problem, other types of drugs may be prescribed: for example diuretics, which lower the resistance in the blood vessels, and beta blockers, which reduce both the heart rate and the amount of blood pumped from the heart with each beat. (Note: asthma sufferers should use beta blockers only with extreme caution, as these drugs can cause spasms in the respiratory passages and lead to breathing difficulties.)

When medication is not sufficient and the individual suffers from severe and recurrent chest pain, surgery may be performed to bypass the major obstructions in the arteries, by creating a detour around the blockage in the artery.

CONGESTIVE HEART FAILURE

Congestive heart failure, often simply called 'heart failure', is a condition in which the heart weakens and fails to keep the blood moving adequately. As a result, the supply of blood to the body's tissues decreases, lowering body efficiency and endurance. With poor circulation, the kidneys fail to remove enough water, salt, and wastes from the blood. In addition, the kidneys, as a result of the decreased blood flow presented to them, also try to increase blood volume by retaining even more salt and water. As a result, blood volume increases, making more work for the already overworked heart, which may enlarge and beat faster in an attempt to satisfy the body's hunger for oxygen-rich blood. Veins distend with fluid and the balance of pressures between fluids inside and outside the veins shifts, which causes fluid that normally stays in the bloodstream to leak into surrounding tissue. This fluid leakage, the reduction of forward blood flow, the backflow of blood, and other factors, are responsible for the accumulation of fluid in the lungs (called pulmonary oedema) as well as for the swelling of the abdomen and legs often seen in patients with congestive heart failure.

CAUSES

The usual cause of congestive heart failure is a diseased heart that just cannot pump enough blood. The most common reason for that is severe coronary artery disease that decreases the flow of blood to the heart muscle. Coronary artery disease is largely responsible for a heart attack, which leaves non-working scar tissue that lowers the efficiency of the heart as a pump. Another important cause is untreated hypertension (high blood pressure), which damages the heart muscle over a period of many years. However, other heart conditions can also cause congestive heart failure. Leaky or narrowed heart valves, due to a birth defect or rheumatic fever, can lead to heart failure. A large cardiac aneurysm, a bulge caused by the thinning of the wall of the lower left heart chamber (ventricle) that pumps blood out of the heart into the body, may weaken the heart's pumping ability.

Less frequently, the root of the problem is one of several different heart muscle diseases. Some are caused by poisons like alcohol, some by viruses, and others by the deposit in the heart tissue of iron or an abnormal body substance known as amyloid. Disturbances of the normal rhythm of the heart may also lead to failure.

SYMPTOMS

Early signs of possible heart failure include unexplained rapid heartbeat, unusual fatigue during exertion, shortness of breath during stair climbing or other mild exercise, and inability to withstand cold. Attacks of shortness of breath and coughing when lying in bed that are relieved by sleeping with pillows under the back to tilt the chest are also early symptoms. Sometimes, a person is actually awakened by 'air hunger' and must sit or stand to breathe more easily. These symptoms are caused by increased fluid pressure in the lung circulation. The relief obtained by assuming a more erect position is due to a shift of fluid (blood) volume to the lower half of the body, easing the burden of the heart. In advanced congestive heart failure, shortness of breath and, frequently, a severe cough with rusty or brownish-coloured sputum (from blood) are common. There may also be swelling of the ankles and a feeling of fullness in the neck or abdomen.

DIAGNOSIS

Usually congestive heart failure can be diagnosed after a physical examination and on the basis of symptoms. However, a chest X-ray is commonly taken to determine how much the heart has become enlarged by its overload and to see if fluid has accumulated within the lungs. In addition, an electro-cardiogram (ECG), a tracing on a graph of the electric current produced by the contraction of the heart muscle, may reveal past heart attack damage and irregularities in the heart rhythm.

TREATMENT

Treatment for congestive heart failure includes rest, oxygen, drugs to strengthen the pumping ability of the heart, and medicine to prevent irregular heart rhythms. Diuretic drugs are given to help the kidneys remove more salt and water from the blood and thus decrease the amount of volume the heart must pump. Recently, doctors have started to prescribe drugs known as ACE inhibitors, for example captopril or enalopril, as these have been shown to improve survival rates in heart failure. They work on the mechanism by which the body controls blood pressure and fluid balance.

In some cases surgery is also done to replace or correct a faulty heart valve, or to repair an aneurysm. Contributing factors to be controlled or eliminated may include high blood pressure, anaemia, excess salt or alcohol intake, fever, over-active thyroid, and stress due to over-exertion.

PREVENTION

Congestive heart failure usually results from an already damaged heart. Thus, the prevention of congestive heart failure rests on those good health habits that help prevent heart disease in general: a well-balanced diet with moderate or low intake of fats; weight control; plenty of exercise, rest, and sleep; avoidance of tobacco and excess alcohol; and periodic medical checkups to detect high blood pressure that might eventually overload or injure the heart and thus lead to congestive heart failure.

In people who already have congestive heart failure, control of the condition is much helped by eliminating highly salted foods, avoiding over-exertion while taking as much exercise as possible, and adhering strictly to the prescribed programme of medication.

CORONARY BYPASS SURGERY

Coronary bypass surgery is performed on one or more of the three great blood vessels, the coronary arteries, that lie on the outer surface of the heart and supply heart muscle with the oxygen and nutrients it needs. In coronary artery disease, a section or sections of the arteries gradually become obstructed with a build-up of cholesterol, calcium, and scar tissue. The purpose of the operation is to bypass the blood around the obstruction using a section of blood vessel (usually a vein taken from the leg) that is sewn into the artery in front of and behind the blockage. This permits free blood flow again. Without it, heart muscle below the obstruction is starved for blood and oxygen, especially during exercise. This creates the chest pains known as 'angina'. If one or more of the coronary arteries become completely obstructed, the result may be a heart attack, in which a portion of heart muscle becomes so starved for blood that it dies.

Usually if there is one obstruction in the coronary arteries, there are others (there may be two in the same artery). A 'double bypass' operation means that two vessels are bypassed, a 'triple bypass' means that three vessels are bypassed, and so forth. Three or more bypasses are common.

Bypass surgery is usually considered when a person suffers frequent chest pains from angina. However, not all persons with angina need bypass surgery. Advances are being made in medication to control angina. Furthermore, some angina is caused by spasms (sudden, violent contractions) of the coronary arteries, which bypass surgery may not prevent or help. Nowadays obstructions in the coronary arteries can sometimes be eliminated by methods that do not require cutting open the chest. This involves crushing the obstruction with a tiny balloon, or burning it with a laser beam that is threaded through the blood vessel from the outside. Even without outside help, and given enough time, the heart creates its own partial bypass, by developing blood vessels that detour the blood around the obstruction; this is known as 'collateral circulation'.

DIAGNOSIS

If you have severe chest pains often and they cannot be controlled by medication, your doctor may decide to order that X-ray motion pictures of your heart be taken. Through a thin woven plastic catheter (tube) entering at the arm or leg and passing through large blood vessels to your heart, X-ray contrast medium is injected so that it flows into the coronary arteries, outlining them on the X-ray screen. The pictures show exactly where the blood vessels are narrowed or blocked. Thus the doctor can determine whether bypasses are needed and where. The most urgent reason to operate is the obstruction, of 50 to 70 per cent or more, of the left-main coronary artery, which supplies two-thirds of the blood to the heart muscle by means of its two lower branches.

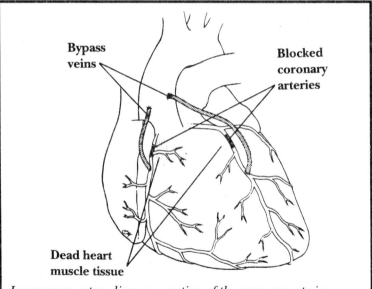

Bypass veins

Blocked coronary arteries

Dead heart muscle tissue

In coronary artery disease, a section of the coronary arteries gradually becomes obstructed with a build-up of cholesterol, calcium, and scar tissue. The coronary bypass operation bypasses the blood around the obstruction in the coronary arteries using a section of blood vessel – usually a vein taken from the leg – that is sewn into the artery in front of and behind the blockage. This permits free blood flow again.

PROCEDURE

The bypass surgery operation takes about four hours or more depending on the number of bypasses. An assisting surgeon cuts several incisions in one leg to obtain a long section of a large vein for use as bypass tubing. Next, the surgeon makes an incision down the middle of the chest, divides the breast-bone with an electric saw, and separates the two sides of the rib cage enough to expose the beating heart. The heartbeat is then stopped using either electric shock, ice water, or drugs. A heart-lung machine, connected to large vessels carrying blood from and to the heart, takes over the job of adding oxygen, removing carbon dioxide, and pumping the blood through the body.

The surgeon cuts through the pericardial sac (a bag of tissue around the heart) to expose the coronary arteries outlined on the heart surface. On either side of each coronary artery blockage, the surgeon cuts open the artery and sews in either end of bypass tube – a piece of vein taken from the leg. Thereafter, blood will flow freely around the obstructed portion to nourish the heart muscle and thereby protect the patient against chest pains and heart attacks. Usually the patient can walk about three or four days following the operation, and return home in little more than a week.

For such a major operation, the death rate is very low – less than 1 per cent in some hospitals. In 80 per cent of cases, angina pains are eliminated and the patient can return to a normal life. Life expectancy may improve but it cannot be guaranteed in all cases.

There has been much controversy surrounding bypass surgery, mainly centring around the question of whether this procedure can increase the life expectancy in those with coronary artery disease and angina. At present, there is no question that the surgery relieves pain and allows for greater exercise tolerance in the majority of patients who undergo it for severe angina.

In certain patterns of disease such as obstruction of the 'left-main' coronary artery, the operation definitely prolongs life expectancy. In other patterns such as 'triple vessel disease' where branches of all three coronaries (except for the left-main) are involved, the surgery most likely allows a longer life. In still other patterns, the question is unsettled. Whether or not the surgery will prevent a heart attack is also an unsettled issue.

EMBOLISM

An embolism occurs when some part of the circulatory system is either partially or completely blocked by some obstructing mass that has travelled through the system. The occurrence of an obstruction is called an *embolism* while the mass causing the embolism is called an *embolus*.

TYPES
Emboli (the plural of embolus) are classified in three major groups:

- Solid emboli, which are made up of a variety of substances, such as clumps of tissue, tumour cells, or pieces of blood clots.
- Liquid emboli, which are made up of globules of fat or amniotic fluid (fluid in which the foetus is bathed during pregnancy).
- Gaseous emboli, which are made up of the different constituents of air.

COMMON LOCATIONS
Emboli are further categorised according to the location of the blockage:

- Arterial emboli, which originate either from the heart or the artery itself, travel downstream, and prevent the flow of fresh blood to whatever area or organ is being supplied.
- Paradoxical emboli, which originate in the venous system and pass over into the arterial system (this usually occurs because of defects in the walls separating the chambers of the heart).

- Pulmonary emboli, which block vessels in the lungs.
- Coronary artery emboli, which block coronary arteries of the heart.
- Cerebral emboli, which usually originate in the heart or the carotid arteries in the neck leading to the brain (these are a major cause of stroke).

CAUSES

Emboli have a variety of causes, depending on the specific type. The most common cause is the breaking away of a blood clot from within the heart or blood vessels. Arterial emboli commonly originate in the heart itself, because of plaques or accumulations on the heart's valves, from blood clots on the walls of the heart, or within an aneurysm. An arterial embolus can also originate from a plaque or clot within the artery itself. Fat emboli can develop from injury to the bones (particularly the long bones of the leg) or from damage to cells in fat tissue. Air emboli can develop (rarely) if a very large amount of air is admitted during an intravenous (into the vein) infusion or as a complication of surgery, especially in operations on the neck or the chest. In these cases, air enters vessels that are open because of the surgery. However, the oxygen in air is not the only gas involved in gaseous emboli. When divers ascend from high pressure levels in the water to normal pressure levels too quickly or when aviators (in planes without cabin pressurisation) climb from normal pressure levels to low pressure levels, there is always the possibility of nitrogen bubbles arising in the bloodstream because of too rapid decompression. If any of these gaseous emboli find their way into the central nervous system, the result can be catastrophic.

An arterial embolism deprives the affected area of its blood supply, which can cause damage or death of the area. An embolism in a brain artery may produce the symptoms of a stroke. In an embolism in the leg, the area beyond the blockage – if totally or nearly totally deprived of blood – becomes white and painful. If the obstruction is not relieved, death of tissue will ensue.

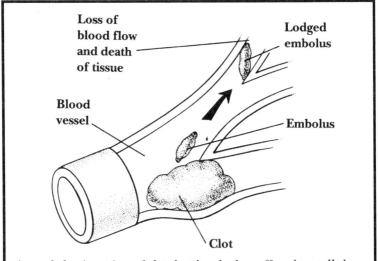

An embolus is a piece of clot that has broken off and travelled through the circulatory system. The embolus will usually lodge downstream causing loss of blood flow and death of tissue in the area nourished by that vessel.

TREATMENT

Emboli resulting from blood clots are often treated with a variety of anticoagulants (agents that inhibit normal clotting mechanisms in the blood). Common anticoagulants such as heparin and warfarin do not actually dissolve clots, but instead prevent additional clots from forming and embolising. There are newer drugs that do dissolve clots, but their use is restricted to special situations. If an embolism is in an available location, such as in an artery in a limb, and tissue is threatened, surgery to remove the clot is the preferred method of treatment to save the limb. In cases of a massive embolism to the lung (usually from deep veins in the legs) where life is threatened, surgery can also be attempted. In addition, if an individual has clots in the deep venous system of the lower half of the body and for some reason (for example, a recent haemorrhage in the brain or other vital organ) anticoagulants cannot be prescribed, blocking devices such as clips can be placed on or in the main vein (inferior vena cava) receiving blood from the lower body to prevent emboli from reaching the lungs.

HEART ATTACK

A heart attack (or myocardial infarction) occurs when an area of the heart muscle is damaged or dies because a coronary artery has been blocked and the oxygen-rich blood supply to that area of the heart has been drastically reduced. The damaged muscle tissue of the heart is replaced with scar tissue, which affects the heart's future performance.

Although the chances of surviving a heart attack are now better than ever and complete recovery is common, heart attack or another form of circulatory disease is still the number one cause of death in this country. Heart attacks that do not result in death often lead to serious complications: shock; cardiac arrhythmia, marked by an irregular heartbeat; or congestive heart failure, in which the heart cannot pump enough blood to meet the body's needs and fluid accumulates in the lower parts of the body.

CAUSES

Heart attack is caused by the total blockage of a coronary artery by a blood clot (thrombus) which forms over an area of atherosclerosis, a disease in which the artery linings become gradually clogged by various fatty deposits, thus shutting off blood flow to the heart. Other healthy arteries that are not clogged may be much narrower and therefore unable to deliver the extra oxygenated blood needed by the heart during emotional stress or physical exertion. So damage to the heart results.

RISK FACTORS

A number of physical and environmental factors, other than a thrombus or atherosclerosis, can increase the chances of heart attack: hypertension (high blood pressure) increases the resistance in the blood vessels, making the heart pump harder to push blood through, although it may actually be less important in causing heart attacks than we used to think. A high level of cholesterol in the blood increases the likelihood

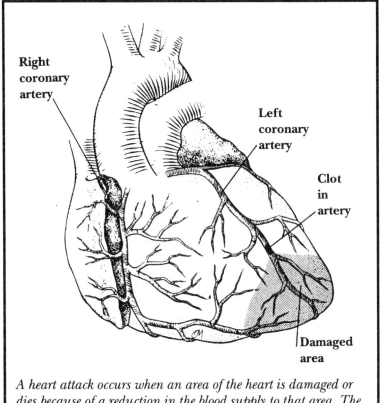

Right coronary artery

Left coronary artery

Clot in artery

Damaged area

A heart attack occurs when an area of the heart is damaged or dies because of a reduction in the blood supply to that area. The reduced blood supply results when the coronary artery supplying the area is blocked by a blood clot or advanced atherosclerosis.

of developing atherosclerosis; and birth control pills, especially those taken by women over the age of 35 or by smokers, have been linked to the increased incidence of heart attack.

Smoking, stress, improper diet, and lack of exercise have also been associated with the increased risk of heart attack. Smoking acts to constrict the arteries and reduce the blood flow to the heart muscle and greatly increases the risk of atherosclerosis. It seems to be the single most important preventable factor in causing heart attacks. Stress probably isn't as important as we used to think, although it puts an extra demand on the heart's need for blood. A diet high in saturated fats (fats that are usually solid at room temperature, including those animal fats found in butter and meats) has been found to increase the serum cholesterol level in the blood and thus the chances of developing atherosclerosis; and the lack of moderate, regular exercise prevents the development of collateral circulation and increases the risk of atherosclerosis. Collateral circulation is the system of smaller blood vessels that bypass a blocked artery and increase the blood supply to the area that the blocked artery serves.

SYMPTOMS

The major symptom of a heart attack is a crushing pain in the middle of the chest, behind the breastbone; the pain can also extend down one or both arms. Fatigue, heavy perspiration, dizziness, difficulty in breathing and, occasionally, fever, may accompany this pain. The pain may be somewhat similar to that experienced from angina pectoris (chest pain), but the pain of a heart attack is more intense, will not be relieved by nitroglycerin, and will not go away within a few minutes, as angina pain will. Also, a heart attack may take place during sleep, which is rare for angina pain.

Heart attacks range from very mild, signalled only by a slight discomfort, faintness and nausea, to very serious, which can be accompanied by cardiac arrest (when the heartbeat completely stops) or ventricular fibrillation (when the normal, steady heartbeat is reduced to a useless quivering that prevents blood from being pumped through the body).

DIAGNOSIS

Heart attack is diagnosed by the electrocardiograph (ECG), which measures the electrical impulses produced by the heart; a diseased heart will show a record of disturbed patterns because the impulses must travel around the damaged area. A test for an increased white blood cell count may also be done, as the body's immune system will increase its number of white blood cells in order to carry away dead tissue from the damaged heart. Other blood tests may be taken to measure certain proteins in the blood that signal damaged heart muscle, although these tests may not show results until 24 to 72 hours after the attack.

TREATMENT

The best and only treatment for heart attack is to rush to a hospital for emergency medical treatment as soon as an attack is suspected. More deaths could be prevented if heart attack victims did not delay going to a hospital. Studies have shown that, on the average, heart attack victims wait three hours before seeing a doctor.

In almost every case, hospitalisation will be necessary following a heart attack. Treatment in the hospital may include care in the cardiac care unit (CCU).

A variety of medications may be used to treat heart attack patients: digitalis, which establishes a steady heartbeat; anti-arrhythmics, which inhibit irregularities in the heartbeat; diuretics, which reduce strain on the heart by removing excess water from the blood; anti-anginals, which diminish chest pain; and beta blockers, which ease the strain on the heart by decreasing its work. But the most important recent advance has been the development of thrombolytic drugs, which can actually dissolve part of the thrombus that is obstructing the coronary artery before too much of the heart muscle is permanently damaged. These drugs are only effective if given as soon as possible, preferably within an hour or two of the attack and certainly within 12 hours. They need to be given by injection, and are generally only given in hospital. This is why it is now more important than ever to seek help without delay.

Lifestyle changes will also help heart attack victims. Patients will be expected to stop smoking, perhaps lose weight, and partake in regular exercise.

PREVENTION

Prevention of heart attack begins with sensible health and dietary habits. Those who do not smoke, do not overeat or overindulge in saturated fats, but do exercise regularly, are much less likely to become heart attack victims. A diet rich in oily fish has been shown to help too. Those who have already suffered one or more heart attacks can prevent further attacks by changes in their living habits along these lines as well as by taking half an aspirin tablet every day, to thin their blood enough to reduce the risk of another thrombus forming. Some may benefit from taking beta blocker tablets to help prevent another heart attack.

HEARTBEAT IRREGULARITIES (ARRHYTHMIA)

Heartbeat irregularities (called arrhythmia) are defined as any deviation from the normal, steady beating of the heart, which is responsible for regular circulation of the blood throughout the body.

Minor irregularities in the heartbeat are common, but more serious arrhythmias can lead to fainting, angina (chest pain), or heart attack. The most devastating heartbeat irregularity is called ventricular fibrillation. This occurs when the normally steady pumping of the heart is reduced to a useless quivering, preventing the heart from pumping sufficient blood throughout the body. Ventricular fibrillation often occurs after a heart attack or some other serious injury, such as a severe electric shock, and it must receive immediate emergency medical attention or it can be fatal.

CAUSES

Arrhythmias are usually caused by damage to the heart muscle or to a small mass of specialised heart tissue called the sinus node. The sinus node, the natural pacemaker of the heart, is responsible for establishing and maintaining a healthy, steady heartbeat.

Heartbeat irregularities can also be caused by improper use of drugs (drugs prescribed for arrhythmia can actually cause it if dosage is too high); excessive smoking (the nicotine in cigarettes slows the heartbeat); or consumption of large quantities of caffeine (the high amounts found in coffee, tea,

157

chocolate, cola, and some cold medicines may overstimulate the heart).

Heartbeat irregularities may also develop as a result of congenital damage (present at birth) to the heart; a poorly functioning left ventricle (the lower chamber of the heart that pumps blood into the arteries); high blood pressure; rheumatic fever; or a previous heart attack in which the resulting scar tissue interferes with the nerve impulses governing the heartbeat.

SYMPTOMS

Some heartbeat irregularities have no noticeable symptoms. Others will be signalled by light-headedness, fainting, a pounding heart, dizziness, and chest pain.

DIAGNOSIS

Arrhythmias are diagnosed primarily with the electrocardiograph (ECG), which records the electrical impulses made by the heart's beating. A normal heart will produce a record of regular peaks and valleys; an arrhythmic heart will show an uneven pattern. Sometimes it may be necessary to wear a small portable ECG recorder for 24 hours or more to catch an occasional arrhythmia.

TREATMENT

Occasionally, an arrhythmia is so mild that no particular treatment is required. But most irregularities are treated with medication, defibrillators, or pacemakers. All of these methods act to steady the irregularities and maintain a healthy, steady heartbeat.

Medications commonly used include digitalis, which slows the heartbeat and is useful for a common arrhythmia called atrial fibrillation; beta blockers, which correct extra beats originating in the lower chambers of the heart; and various antiarrhythmics, which act on specific problems of the heartbeat.

A defibrillator is a device applied to the chest which electrically jolts the quivering heart that is suffering from ventricular fibrillation back into a normal pattern of beating.

For those whose arrhythmia is caused by a faulty sinus node, an artificial pacemaker may be implanted in the heart. A pacemaker is a tiny electrical device powered by a small generator which, when implanted in the chest, acts to steady an abnormal heartbeat. Once inserted under the skin and threaded through a vein into the heart, it takes over the job of regulating the heartbeat by sending out electrical impulses similar to those emitted by the heart. Some pacemakers only go into action when the heart fails to beat after a specified time period; others completely take over the heart's job and are set to beat at a constant rate, usually about 72 times per minute.

Lifestyle changes will probably be recommended to patients suffering from heartbeat irregularities; they may need to stop smoking, lose weight, exercise more regularly, and reduce their caffeine intake. These precautions may also be taken in an effort to prevent arrhythmias.

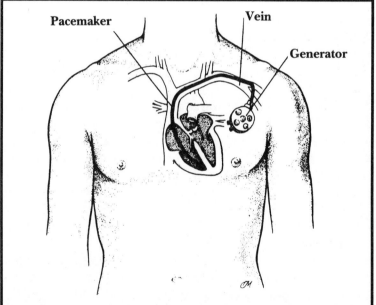

Pacemaker   **Vein**

Generator

A mechanical pacemaker, a tiny electrical device powered by a small generator, can be used to correct heartbeat irregularities in people whose natural pacemaker is defective. The pacemaker is inserted into the chest and threaded through a vein until it rests within the heart. The generator is then sewn under the skin.

HEART MURMURS

Heart murmurs are extra whishing sounds – over and above the regular 'lub-dub' sound of the heartbeat – made as blood flows through heart valves.

Heart murmurs can be congenital (existing at birth but not hereditary) or acquired because of rheumatic fever, atherosclerosis, syphilis, or other ailments.

INNOCENT HEART MURMURS

Heart murmurs can be heard in many healthy people, especially children, teenagers, and pregnant women, and in these cases are considered innocent or functional because they are a normal sound caused by the blood rushing through the heart.

ABNORMAL HEART MURMURS

On the other hand, heart murmurs can be a symptom that first alerts a doctor to the possibility of a heart condition or disease.

These abnormal murmurs come from vibrations or turbulence in the bloodstream. They are called organic or structural heart murmurs and can be caused by blood being forced through narrowed or obstructed heart valves, a defect in the heart walls, or valves that do not close completely and allow blood to seep back into the upper or lower heart chambers.

SYMPTOMS

Heart murmurs can be detected only by physical examination. A doctor listening to the heart through a stethoscope can usually distinguish any extra sound and identify whether or not it signifies a serious problem by its quality, intensity, location and timing.

DIAGNOSIS AND TREATMENT

A person with a functional or innocent heart murmur can live a completely normal life. If the heart murmur is organic or structural, the doctor will order tests (chest X-ray, electrocardiogram, ultrasound, cardiac catheterisation, echocardiogram, or fluoroscopy) to evaluate the extent of the condition and prescribe appropriate treatment. Some people with heart murmurs must take antibiotics before any dental or surgical procedure, even if minor, because of an increased risk of infection of their heart valves.

HAEMORRHAGE

Haemorrhage is the technical term for bleeding, often referring to substantial blood loss or uncontrollable bleeding, either externally or internally. The effects of and damage from haemorrhage depend on the part of the body that is bleeding and the total amount of blood that is lost. Haemorrhage can be a symptom of a number of serious, sometimes fatal, disorders.

CAUSES

Haemorrhage occurs when blood vessels are torn or broken. In normal situations, blood clots within seconds or minutes, stopping the blood flow. However, when serious injuries or other disorders are involved, the body's normal blood-clotting function may be inadequate or malfunctioning; if blood loss is not quickly stopped, death may result.

When the blood-clotting mechanism is temporarily inadequate (usually caused by some kind of serious injury) or when the blood-clotting mechanism has been disrupted as a result of some disorder (including haemophilia, thrombocytopaenia, peptic ulcer, cancer, or diseases involving the stomach, kidney, or urinary tract), internal haemorrhage may result.

161

SYMPTOMS

Severe external haemorrhage displays the following symptoms: rapid pulse; dizziness or faintness; collapse; shock; a drop in blood pressure and a rise in pulse rate; and pale, cold, clammy, or sweaty skin.

Internal haemorrhage may also show symptoms, even if the bleeding is slight. Black, tarry stools may signal bleeding in the intestinal tract from a peptic ulcer or cancer of the colon; blood in the vomitus indicates bleeding in the stomach; and blood in the urine means bleeding is occurring in the kidneys or urinary tract.

Blood in the stool, urine, or vomitus should always be reported to a doctor at once, as should external bleeding that occurs frequently or that cannot be stopped within minutes or hours, depending on the severity of the wound.

TREATMENT

Treatment for internal haemorrhage involves correcting the cause of the bleeding, possibly with surgery. External haemorrhage is treated by applying pressure to the wound with a sterile bandage (or, in an emergency, just pressing it with the fingers) until the bleeding stops. If bleeding cannot be stopped, the patient will almost certainly be hospitalised, where lost blood can be replaced with blood transfusions or damaged blood vessels can be surgically tied off and sealed.

HYPERTENSION

Hypertension, or high blood pressure, refers to persistently elevated pressure of blood within and against the walls of the arteries, which carry blood from the heart through the body. This excessive force being exerted on the artery walls may cause damage to the arteries themselves and thereby to body organs such as the heart, kidney, and brain, leading to heart attacks, kidney failure, and strokes.

CAUSES

Although many people believe hypertension is a condition caused by extreme activity or tension, this is not so. Actually, high blood pressure may have no known cause, or it can be associated with other diseases. When no underlying cause is discovered, the disease is called primary or essential hypertension. If another disease, such as kidney or heart disease, causes the elevated blood pressure, the condition is labelled secondary hypertension.

Contrary to popular belief, there is no typical hypertensive person. However, there are some people more susceptible to developing high blood pressure. Persons with either one or both parents who are hypertensive are at greater risk of acquiring this condition since heredity may play a role in the development of hypertension. In the past, hypertension has been attributed to ageing, but current evidence shows that age is not a primary factor. Black people, both children and adults, have at least twice the incidence of hypertension as white people.

Overweight, heavy drinking, and excessive sodium (salt) in the diet causing fluid retention may increase blood pressure, especially in people prone to hypertension. There are also indications that oral contraceptives may contribute to increased blood pressure. However, this is more likely to occur with women who are overweight, whose parents are hypertensive, or who have other hypertensive risk factors.

SYMPTOMS

Hypertension has been called the 'silent disease', because it often has no obvious symptoms. A person may have high blood pressure for years without noticing any symptoms. Rare symptoms may include headache, ear ringing, thumping in the chest, or possibly frequent nosebleeds. However, these symptoms may result from other conditions.

DIAGNOSIS

To diagnose hypertension, a simple, risk-free, painless test using a stethoscope and a sphygmomanometer, an inflatable arm cuff attached to a graduated mercury manometer (device measuring the tension of fluids), is used. Blood pressure is measured in a main artery of the arm by first shutting off and then releasing the flow of blood in the artery with the cuff and listening to the artery pulse with the stethoscope.

The blood pressure measurements are read as the systolic pressure (the first beat of the pulse after release of the cuff) over the diastolic pressure (the pressure at which the last beat is heard) – for example, 120/80 is considered normal in the average adult. The systolic pressure essentially measures the pressure of the heart during a contraction or heartbeat. The diastolic pressure is that which exists when the heart is filling between beats. Although diastolic pressure is considerably lower than systolic, there is still pressure in the body when the heart is filling. Therefore, both numbers count. An unusually high systolic pressure may mean the heart is pumping too hard or the arteries are stiff; a high diastolic pressure means that the arteries have an abnormally high tone or resistance.

Normal blood pressure is about 80/46 at birth and climbs as age increases. The normal adult pressure is around 120/80. Female hypertensives seem to do better than males; however, their risk of cardiovascular disease is still greater than that of normal females.

TREATMENT

Fortunately, hypertension responds well to treatment. When the condition is mild (systolic around 140 and diastolic up to 100) and there is no indication of other disease, doctors may suggest lifestyle changes before prescribing medication. These changes may include weight loss for the overweight and a regular exercise program. Heavy drinkers should cut down, and smokers should try to stop. Although smoking doesn't increase the risk of hypertension, it does increase the risk of complication from it.

If medication is indicated, a doctor may prescribe one drug or a combination of drugs as part of a 'stepped care' pro-gramme. Step one may start with a diuretic, a drug that promotes water loss. Step two may be a beta blocker, a medi-cine that reduces the work of the heart, or occasionally a 'centrally acting' drug that lowers blood pressure by affecting the blood pressure centre of the brain. Step three could be a vasodilator, a drug that dilates or opens narrowed blood vessels that contribute to hypertension by increasing resistance to flow. If none of the first three steps proves effective, a combination of two or more steps may be repeated or other still more potent drugs may be used – all under the doctor's close supervision.

While tension and stress do not directly cause hypertension, these factors do affect the condition. Persons with hypertension are urged to avoid high-pressure situations and learn to deal with stress. Since techniques such as biofeedback, self-hypnosis, and meditation have proven useful for reducing stress, they may help someone with hypertension. Blood pressure can be monitored at home by purchasing a special kit and learning to use the sphygmomanometer. Children of hypertensive parents especially need to have their blood pressure measured early in life on a regular basis. If three separate elevated readings (above 140/90 in adults) are detected, a trip to the doctor is in order. Cutting down on dietary salt can help to reduce blood pressure, but only if salt restriction is so extreme that most food is bland or even unpalatable. Drugs are more effective, and usually have fewer side effects.

STROKE

Stroke is an interruption of the blood supply to a group of brain cells, damaging those cells and causing malfunction or lack of function in those parts of the body that the damaged cells control. Generally speaking, each side of the brain controls the motor and sensory functions of the opposite side of the body, so damage to cells on the left side of the brain, for instance, will impair function on the right side of the body.

Stroke can have a wide range of consequences; it may, among other conditions, cause temporary or permanent loss of memory and difficulty in speaking, walking, and controlling emotions.

CAUSES

Stroke can be caused by several conditions. One is called cerebrovascular embolism, which occurs when a 'wandering' blood clot, formed elsewhere in the body (usually in the heart or in one or both carotid arteries in the neck that carry blood from the heart to the brain), lodges itself in an artery leading to or within the brain. Interruption of blood flow also occurs when a similar clot is formed in the arteries because of the presence of atherosclerosis (a narrowing and clogging of the arteries by various deposits).

Stroke can also be caused by cerebral haemorrhage, in which a diseased artery in the brain bursts, depriving the cells that are normally nourished by that artery, as well as flooding the surrounding tissue with blood. This accumulation of blood forms a clot which displaces and compresses brain tissue and thus interferes in the brain's functioning. This type of stroke often strikes people who have both hypertension (high blood pressure) and atherosclerosis.

A third condition that can lead to stroke may be an aneurysm (a bulge in an artery because of a defect in its wall) that ruptures and interrupts blood flow to an area of the brain as well as flooding the area with blood. The formation of aneurysms is sometimes associated with hypertension, but is often congenital (present at birth). Thus aneurysms are often the cause of cerebral haemorrhage in young people.

THOSE AT RISK

People who have both hypertension and atherosclerosis are the most likely to suffer a stroke, since both diseases weaken and damage the arteries. Hypertension probably encourages haemorrhage. Heredity may play a role in stroke, since the tendencies to develop both hypertension and atherosclerosis appear to be inherited. Black people are more likely candidates for stroke because high blood pressure is at least twice as common among black people as among white.

Smoking, diabetes, and high blood cholesterol may also contribute to stroke. Furthermore, stroke is more likely to victimise anyone with a history of mild stroke-like episodes called TIAs (transient ischaemic attacks). TIAs are essentially strokes that clear up within 24 hours, that is, an individual may develop paralysis of one side of the body as in a classic stroke, but the symptoms clear within 24 hours, leaving no residual effects.

SYMPTOMS
A stroke can present itself in many ways, but some of the more common symptoms are a sudden weakness or numbness in the face, arm and/or leg on one side of the body; loss or slurring of speech or difficulty in understanding others speak; unexplained unsteadiness, and persistent falling to one side. It is possible, however, to suffer a mild stroke and experience minor degrees of these symptoms.

DIAGNOSIS
Stroke is diagnosed mostly by the history and physical examination. Sophisticated X-ray techniques are also employed. For example, arteriography (the injection of X-ray opaque dye into a main artery) will show damage or clots in the arteries leading to or within the brain, and a computerised axial tomography (CAT) scan produces a cross-sectional picture of the area, which can provide the doctor with crucial information such as whether the stroke was caused by a haemorrhage or by blockage of blood flow. Tumours, which can cause symptoms identical to that of stroke, are also frequently diagnosed by these means.

TREATMENT
Blood pressure is brought under control if it is high, and drug therapy, to prevent further damage as well as to reduce swelling of the brain tissue, is often instituted. Also, depending on the cause of the stroke and other factors, anticoagulants (agents that inhibit the normal clotting of blood) such as aspirin, are sometimes administered in the hope of limiting the progress of the stroke or preventing additional strokes. After the acute period, rehabilitation is begun by speech, physical, and occupational therapists.

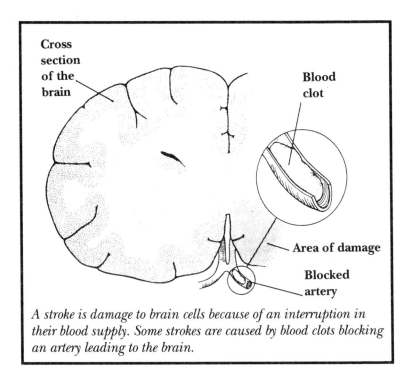

Cross section of the brain

Blood clot

Area of damage

Blocked artery

A stroke is damage to brain cells because of an interruption in their blood supply. Some strokes are caused by blood clots blocking an artery leading to the brain.

PREVENTION

For those who have experienced TIAs or other warning signs of stroke, precautions can be taken to prevent an actual stroke. Sometimes after a TIA, some form of arteriography is performed to locate obstructions or ulcerated areas of the carotid arteries. Depending on the results of the arteriogram along with the general condition of the patient and many other factors, the decision of whether to operate (to 'clean out' the arteries) or to treat with anticoagulants is made. All patients with TIAs may benefit from taking half an aspirin tablet every day. This thins the blood enough to reduce the risk of a stroke.

Other risk factors such as smoking and high cholesterol intake need to be controlled too.

THROMBOPHLEBITIS

Thrombophlebitis is a condition in which both inflammation and blood clots exist in a vein. This can be caused by a number of factors. Commonly, when a person is immobilised, blood stagnates in the veins of the legs; this induces clotting which in turn prevents blood from returning to the heart. The blood below the clot remains there, causing a build-up of pressure that forces fluid into the tissues thus resulting in swelling. Also, simultaneously, the vein(s) and surrounding area may become quite inflamed and tender. This condition is most often found in the deep veins of the legs, but it can also occur in veins of the pelvis and arms.

Thrombophlebitis itself may not be too serious, but it can lead to a life-threatening condition called pulmonary embolism (a blood clot lodged in the lung). This develops when a clot formed in a deep leg vein breaks loose, travels through the bloodstream, and becomes lodged in the vessels of the lung. A pulmonary embolism can lead to chest pain, shortness of breath, coughing up of blood, and even death.

CAUSES

The development of thrombophlebitis is favoured by any condition that inhibits the free flow of blood through the veins. These include prolonged bed rest or inactivity, perhaps following illness or surgery; congestive heart failure, which affects the heart's ability to pump blood throughout the body; and injury or infection that damages a vein. Other factors that may lead to an increased tendency toward thrombophlebitis are the use of birth control pills in susceptible individuals, as well as pregnancy itself; occupations that require long periods of standing or sitting; obesity; old age; and chronic infections. In addition, thrombophlebitis, in some cases, may indicate the presence of a tumour in the pancreas or lung, since these disorders might produce or release a substance that affects blood clotting.

SYMPTOMS

Common symptoms (which often appear only in advanced cases) of deep thrombophlebitis are swelling, aching, and a feeling of heaviness in the leg or affected area; the skin may appear white, or hot and red, and will be painful to the touch. If the veins of the leg are affected, the condition is characterised by increased pain when walking or when the foot is flexed backward or forward.

DIAGNOSIS

Thrombophlebitis of a surface vein (known as superficial thrombophlebitis) can be diagnosed by a simple physical examination usually revealing a red, warm, tender cord-like vein. Superficial thrombophlebitis rarely, if ever, leads to pulmonary embolism.

Diagnostic tests for thrombophlebitis include the Doppler (a technique used to detect obstructions by changes in sounds made by flowing blood), nuclear scans, a test to measure the resistance to flow in the veins, and venography. Venography involves the insertion of X-ray contrast dye into the veins so that the X-ray will visualise a clot. This is the most sensitive and specific test for thrombophlebitis.

TREATMENT

Treatment of superficial thrombophlebitis consists of anti-inflammatory painkillers, and elastic stockings if the legs are involved.

Deep vein thrombophlebitis, because of the potential for pulmonary embolism, is treated much more aggressively. The patient is usually hospitalised and put on bed rest with the leg elevated. The anticoagulant (an anticoagulant is an agent that inhibits the normal clotting mechanisms of the blood) heparin is given intravenously, usually for about seven days, and up to ten days if pulmonary embolism has occurred. The patient is also usually placed on the oral anticoagulant warfarin for about six weeks, or three to six months if pulmonary embolism has occurred. It is important to note that these drugs do not dissolve an existing clot, but serve to prevent new clots from forming while the old ones are resolving. Newer

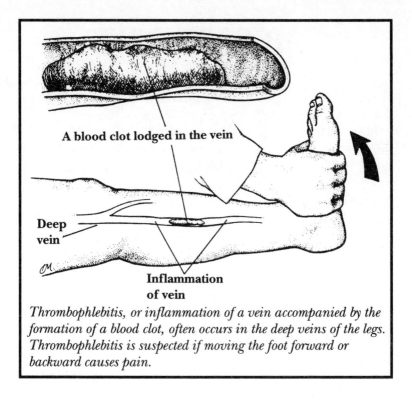

A blood clot lodged in the vein

**Deep
vein**

**Inflammation
of vein**

*Thrombophlebitis, or inflammation of a vein accompanied by the
formation of a blood clot, often occurs in the deep veins of the legs.
Thrombophlebitis is suspected if moving the foot forward or
backward causes pain.*

drugs do dissolve clots, but are still used only in special
situations.

PREVENTION

Prevention of thrombophlebitis is a controversial subject. In
hospitalised patients who are immobilised for long periods or
about to undergo major surgery, leg exercises along with long
support stockings and increased activity as soon as feasible
may be helpful. So-called 'mini-heparin' (low doses of heparin
given by injection under the skin two to three times a day) has
also been beneficial in preventing deep vein thrombophlebitis in certain patients. For patients at home who are
susceptible to this condition, regular exercise of the legs along
with elevation of legs when lying down and support hose are
probably helpful. Self-injected heparin and warfarin are also
used.

VARICOSE VEINS

Varicose veins are swollen, stretched veins in the legs, close to the surface of the skin, caused by pooling of blood.

Blood from the legs needs to return uphill, against the force of gravity, to the heart, so the veins in the legs are lined with one-way valves to prevent blood from flowing back down toward the feet. When pressure on the veins stretches them, the valves cannot close properly, and some blood travels back down. This blood accumulates in pools, which stretch the veins even more. The result is varicose veins, highly visible bluish lines that bulge from the legs and that can be very painful.

Varicose veins alone are not too serious, but they may lead to other conditions: a leg ulcer (an eroded patch on the skin); phlebitis (an inflamed vein); or a blood clot (a thrombus).

CAUSES

Possible causes of varicose veins may include a number of factors that put excess pressure on the veins in the legs: prolonged standing; prolonged sitting, especially with the legs crossed; lack of exercise; confining clothes; a diet low in fibre (hard stools and the pressure needed to excrete them put extra stress on the veins); obesity (which puts excess pressure on the legs and contributes to the muscles' inability to push blood upward); heredity (a tendency toward weak vein walls and valves seems to be inherited); and even height (tall people may be more likely to develop this condition because their blood needs to travel farther in its return trip to the heart).

Pregnancy greatly contributes to the development of varicose veins because female hormones, especially those released at this time, tend to relax the walls of the veins. Thus, the condition is more commonly seen in women than in men. Varicose veins often appear during the last few months of pregnancy due to the increased strain from the weight of the growing uterus. These veins may recede after the baby is born.

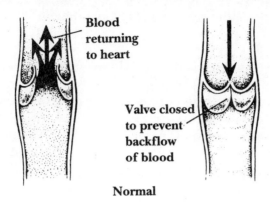

Blood returning to heart

Valve closed to prevent backflow of blood

Normal

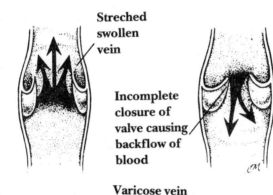

Streched swollen vein

Incomplete closure of valve causing backflow of blood

Varicose vein

At top, the illustration shows the interior of a normal vein, in which blood returning to the heart is not allowed to drop downward by the action of the valve. In the bottom drawing, the vein's valve has been weakened and cannot completely close, thus resulting in an accumulation of excess blood in the vein. The result is a varicose vein.

SYMPTOMS

Varicose veins are very noticeable since they form close to the skin. They appear as bulging, bluish, cord-like lines running down the legs. Symptoms that accompany varicose veins are feelings of achiness, heaviness, and fatigue in the legs, especially at the end of the day; itchy, scaly skin covering the

173

affected areas; and, in advanced cases, swollen ankles, pain shooting down the leg, and leg cramps at night.

TREATMENT

Varicose veins are usually treated by wearing elastic stockings, which act like muscles to help push the blood upward. Severe cases may require a surgical procedure called vein stripping, in which the afflicted veins are tied off and removed; other healthy veins in the area will take over the job of pushing blood toward the heart. A chemical can also be injected into the veins, closing them off and forcing the blood to find other channels to the heart.

Those with varicose veins may need to lose weight, increase the fibre in their diets, exercise regularly, and stretch their legs or put their feet up whenever possible. Exercises to improve circulation in the legs, such as standing on tip-toe, may help relieve pressure.

The Digestive System

Digestion is the process whereby the body converts food into basic substances that can either be absorbed in the bloodstream as nutrients or passed out of the body as waste. This breakdown and assimilation occurs within the digestive tract, a convoluted tube over 30 feet long lined by a mucous membrane that aids in absorbing nutrients.

The tract includes several hollow organs – mouth, oesophagus, stomach, small intestine, and large intestine (colon) – each of which has a specific function in digestion. Muscles of these organs move the food through the system while mucus lubricates the tract and prevents irritation. Solid organs – the liver, gall bladder, and pancreas – also are critical in digestion.

Food first enters the digestive tract through the mouth. In the mouth, the jaws and teeth chew the food into smaller pieces that are mixed with saliva, a secretion of the salivary glands in the mouth. Saliva moistens food for easier swallowing and contains an enzyme (a special protein) that begins breakdown of starches.

From the mouth, food passes down the throat and into the oesophagus (a muscular tube) through which it is conducted to the stomach. The stomach is a large pouch or sac in the abdominal cavity where food is combined with acid and digestive juices secreted by gastric glands within the stomach. The food becomes semi-fluid so that it can pass into the small intestine.

In the first ten inches (duodenum) of the small intestine, food is broken down further with additional digestive juices from the liver and pancreas. This process further separates

175

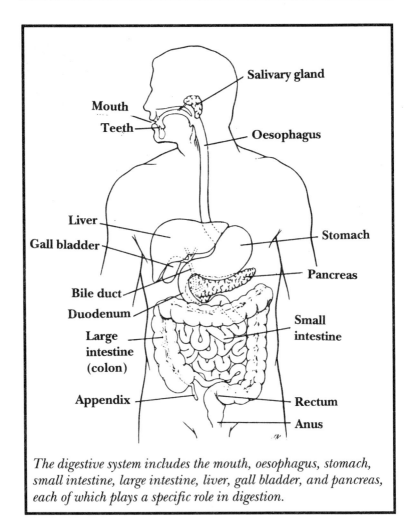

The digestive system includes the mouth, oesophagus, stomach, small intestine, large intestine, liver, gall bladder, and pancreas, each of which plays a specific role in digestion.

nutrients and allows for their absorption into the bloodstream, which takes place in the remainder of the small intestine.

Aiding digestion is the liver, an accessory organ of digestion. The liver produces bile that is necessary for absorption of fat in the small intestine. The liver also functions to purify and remove some wastes from the blood, as well as to produce and store glucose and to process many drugs.

176

The gall bladder on the underside of the liver is another organ that provides an indirect digestive function. The gall bladder stores the bile manufactured by the liver. As bile is needed, the gall bladder contracts and releases the fluid into the small intestine.

Other digestive juices required by the small intestine to digest and absorb food, particularly fats and starches, come from the pancreas, an organ located just under the stomach. The pancreas also secretes insulin and other hormones into the blood. Insulin is the hormone responsible for aiding absorption and use of glucose (sugar).

Whatever substances are not assimilated into the bloodstream through the small intestine move into the large intestine. Within the large intestine, waste material is processed into stool (faeces). At this point, too, water is absorbed to preserve the body's balance of fluids.

The left colon then stores the faecal matter until its transfer to the rectum, its lower part. Once in the rectum, waste is ready to be passed out of the body through the opening at the end of the digestive tract (anus), thus completing the cycle of digestion.

APPENDICITIS

Appendicitis is an inflammation of the appendix that results from a bacterial infection.

The appendix is a small wormlike portion of intestinal tissue located at the juncture of the small and large intestines. Although it may have had a function at some point in human development, the appendix serves no purpose now.

CAUSES

Nevertheless, despite its uselessness, the appendix can cause problems when it becomes inflamed. Inflammation occurs when the hollow tubular structure clogs with masses of waste matter, intestinal worms, or other material that can prevent normal drainage. The blockage provides a fertile environment for bacteria to grow and multiply, thereby causing infection and inflammation.

SYMPTOMS

In the beginning, appendicitis may produce a dull or sharp pain in the navel area of the abdomen. Any movement, coughing or sneezing can intensify the pain. Patients in early stages may also feel nauseous and be unable to eat. Constipation usually accompanies appendicitis; nonetheless about 10 per cent of the patients may have diarrhoea instead. Adults may run a mild fever (up to 39°C), but children generally experience higher fevers. Occasionally, pulse rates accelerate to about 100 beats per minute.

Within hours, the pain becomes continuous and moves to the lower right side of the abdomen over the appendix. Because the location of the appendix may vary depending upon the individual, pain may emanate from the back, side, or pelvis, or even the opposite side of the abdomen. The entire appendix area becomes extremely tender as abdominal muscles tighten.

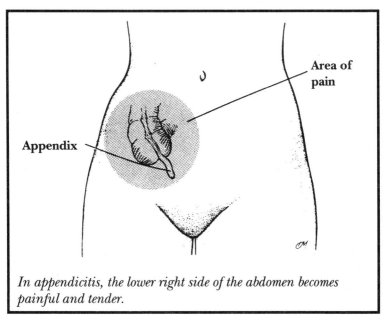

In appendicitis, the lower right side of the abdomen becomes painful and tender.

If fever rises and pain grows more intense, chances of rupture become greater. Rupture results when the appendix becomes so swollen and filled with pus from bacteria that it bursts, spreading infection to surrounding organs. Infection spreads so quickly that gangrene of the appendix may occur within hours after the first symptoms. One serious complication of rupture is peritonitis, an inflammation of the lining of the abdominal cavity.

Any fever with nausea and abdominal pain should be reported to a doctor. Appendicitis is a medical emergency that must be diagnosed to prevent potentially fatal complications. It can affect anyone, but is more prevalent among people between ten and 30 years of age.

DIAGNOSIS

When confirming appendicitis, the doctor checks for tenderness over the appendix. A blood test determines whether or not there is a high white blood cell count (with an infection, the body produces extra white blood cells to help fight the disease). Moreover, the doctor may perform additional tests to rule out other diseases sometimes mistaken for appendicitis, such as gall bladder attack, kidney stones, or kidney infection. In women a twisted ovarian cyst (growth on the female sex organ) or a ruptured ectopic (tubal) pregnancy, may produce symptoms similar to those of appendicitis.

TREATMENT

Although appendicitis cannot be prevented, prompt diagnosis can lead to effective treatment. Patients who suspect appendicitis should not eat food or drink water, or take drugs to relieve pain until a doctor is consulted. Eating or drinking any substance, including laxatives, may cause the appendix to rupture by stimulating activity in the intestine.

A mild case of appendicitis may subside by itself, but it is not worth taking the risk. The cure for acute appendicitis is surgery to remove the inflamed organ and to avoid complications. To insure against further infection, antibiotics may also be prescribed.

CIRRHOSIS

Cirrhosis is a disease in which the cells throughout the liver are progressively destroyed. They are replaced by nodules (swellings) containing normal new cells but also by much connective tissue that alters the structure of the organ. The flow of blood and lymph through the damaged liver is much less efficient, and eventually the liver fails.

CAUSES

Cirrhosis is the liver's attempt to rebuild itself and continue despite injury – from whatever cause. The injury may be a sudden and massive infection, as from hepatitis. It may occur in a less severe manner over months or years, as in chronic active hepatitis or in obstruction of the bile ducts within the liver. The latter process starts with inflammation, then scarring, then closure of the ducts. A similar condition is caused by obstruction of external bile ducts by a stone, scar, inborn defect, or tumour. The damage may be done over an even longer time, slowly and steadily, by alcohol abuse.

Alcoholism is by far the most common cause of cirrhosis. Once thought to be due to the poisonous effect of alcohol on the liver, its damage is now believed to result chiefly from malnutrition. Alcoholics get most of their calories from alcohol and so their diets are dangerously unbalanced. Lack of protein in the diet of an alcoholic, for example, causes scarring in a vital area of the liver. Other causes include:

- Some powerful medications – chemicals such as methotrexate, an anti-cancer drug; halothane, an anaesthetic; and oxyphenisatin, a medicine used in enemas – may also cause liver damage.
- Inborn errors in physical or chemical processes of the body.
- Syphilis.
- Passive liver congestion caused by a clot blocking the large (hepatic) vein carrying blood to the heart, or by an inefficient heart that cannot accept a normal flow of blood from the liver.

SYMPTOMS

Frequently, cirrhosis is not suspected until it is well advanced, for it imitates many other diseases. Symptoms include a general weakness, a vague sick feeling, loss of appetite, loss of weight, and a loss of interest in sex. There may be a dull abdominal ache, nausea, constipation, or diarrhoea. In a malnourished patient, the tongue may be inflamed. Many symptoms are the result of high blood pressure in the portal vein, which brings nutrient-bearing blood from the intestinal area to the liver where the blood is processed. In cirrhosis, the liver cannot handle a normal flow of blood, so the pressure in the portal vein rises. One result is that fluid from the blood is lost into the abdominal cavity. The fluid build-up may press against the diaphragm (the muscular wall separating the abdominal and chest cavities) and interfere with breathing. New blood vessels (collateral vessels) form to carry away the excess blood into the general circulation. There may be bleeding in the oesophagus (food pipe) or stomach, when new collateral vessels burst under pressure. The patient may vomit blood. Serious, life-threatening haemorrhage may occur.

Other symptoms include an enlarged, firm liver and enlarged spleen; a mottled redness of the mound of the palm at the base of the thumb; 'spider veins' on the skin of the upper body; loss of hair from chest and pubic area; diminishing testicles; and tingling sensations on the skin of the hands and feet.

DIAGNOSIS

Proof of cirrhosis of the liver is furnished by liver biopsy. A hollow needle is inserted through the skin and into the liver itself to obtain a tissue sample for analysis. Tissue from a diseased liver reveals destruction of cells and scarring. Other diagnostic procedures include radionuclide scanning (in this procedure, the patient takes in traces of radioactive material that travels to the liver and illuminates a picture of the organ onto the screen of the scanner). X-ray pictures are taken of the gall bladder and of bile ducts inside the liver and leading from it. Blood and urine tests reveal important clues, including bile pigments in the blood, low red blood cell count, vitamin and mineral deficiencies, and protein in the urine.

TREATMENT

Treatment aims first to remove the cause of the original injury. Thus an alcoholic patient needs to stop drinking, is placed on a well-balanced moderate-to-high-protein diet, and is given larger than usual doses of multivitamins (supplemental vitamins include A, B complex, D, and K – which cannot be stored in the ill liver – and folic acid). If a stone is obstructing an external bile duct and thus causing liver damage, it can be removed. Diuretic drugs may be needed to reduce fluid build-up in the body. Good care includes plenty of rest and frequent small meals, rather than fewer large ones, to reduce the work load on the liver, and avoiding any infection that might cause new stress on the liver.

PREVENTION

Drinking moderately is the best way to reduce the risk of developing this serious disease. Safe upper limits seem to be around 14 units of alcohol a week for a woman, and 21 for a man. A unit of alcohol is equivalent to a glass of wine, a single measure of spirits, or a half-pint of beer.

COLITIS AND IRRITABLE BOWEL

Colitis is a general term meaning an inflammation of the colon (large intestine). It is usually a chronic (long-term) condition that is characterised by sudden attacks followed by periods of remission (relief). It should not be confused with irritable bowel syndrome (also called spastic colon), which is not an inflammation of the colon. Irritable bowel syndrome, or IBS, causes bouts of pain in the lower abdomen, often on the left side. There may be diarrhoea, or constipation, or often alternating bouts of both. The symptoms are due to excessive activity of the muscles in the lower part of the bowel. The cause is unknown, although stress, and a diet without much fibre, often trigger attacks. Treatment includes a high-fibre diet, drugs to relax the over-active bowel, and hypnotherapy to counteract stress.

Frequently, the term colitis is used synonymously with an entity known as 'inflammatory bowel disease'. There are basically three diseases incorporated under this term: ulcerative colitis, Crohn's disease (regional or granulomatous colitis), and ulcerative proctitis. Ulcerative colitis involves only the large intestine (except in rare instances). Crohn's disease may involve any portion of the food tract, including the mouth, and on occasion may not involve the colon. Ulcerative proctitis, the least serious of the group, involves only the rectum, but can closely resemble ulcerative colitis.

CAUSES
In some cases, the cause of colitis is unknown, although it can be a result of a bacterial infection or, in older people, lack of blood to the colon.

SYMPTOMS
Colitis may begin slowly with abdominal discomfort, mild diarrhoea or constipation, and a general feeling of being unwell. As the condition becomes more severe, symptoms such as abdominal pain or bleeding from the rectum may appear. If the disease appears suddenly, the patient may experience fever, bloody diarrhoea, loss of appetite, and weight loss.

DIAGNOSIS
The diagnosis of colitis is based on a direct inspection of intestinal walls with the aid of a sigmoidoscope (or proctoscope), a lighted tube inserted into the colon through the anus, the opening to the outside of the body. A tissue sample of the intestinal wall may be taken to be examined under the microscope. Other tests may be done to rule out other diseases or disorders of the colon.

TREATMENT

People with a mild case of colitis can usually be treated at home and be permitted a normal diet. More seriously ill patients may be treated in the hospital with a special diet to allow the digestive tract to rest; replacement (often intra-venously) of fluids and salts lost during episodes of diarrhoea and/or bleeding; and medications, for example, antibiotics to treat an infection or cortisone (and other drugs) to treat inflammatory bowel disease. Those individuals with severe cases of colitis may require blood transfusions and perhaps even surgery to remove the inflamed portion of the colon.

DIABETES MELLITUS

Diabetes mellitus, often called sugar diabetes, is a condition in which the body is unable to process properly carbohydrates (sug-ars and starches), which are the body's major source of energy.

Normally, digestion causes these carbohydrates to release a form of sugar called glucose into the blood. As the blood glucose level rises, the pancreas gland located in the upper abdomen is stimulated to secrete the hormone insulin. Insulin acts to reduce the sugar content in the blood by transporting glucose from the blood to body cells where it is used for fuel or to the liver where it is stored until needed for fuel.

When the pancreas produces insufficient insulin or the body cannot use the insulin it manufactures, diabetes results. Sugar concentrations accumulate in the blood as glucose circulates throughout the body without being absorbed. Even-tually, the kidney filters sugar from the blood, and urine (the fluid mixture of water and waste products) carries the excess blood sugar from the body.

TYPES

There are two major forms of diabetes. Type I, or insulin-dependent, diabetes results from a defect of unknown origin in the islets of Langerhans, the part of the pancreas that

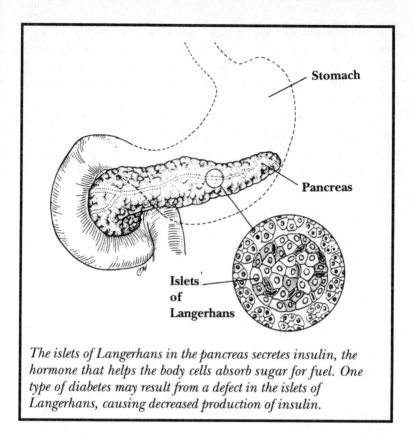

The islets of Langerhans in the pancreas secretes insulin, the hormone that helps the body cells absorb sugar for fuel. One type of diabetes may result from a defect in the islets of Langerhans, causing decreased production of insulin.

produces insulin. This form of diabetes can develop in very young children.

With Type II, or insulin-independent, diabetes the pancreas functions adequately, but the body is unable to use insulin efficiently. Sometimes, a shortage of insulin-receptor cells (sites throughout the body where interaction of sugar and insulin occurs) allows the insulin to float in the bloodstream without working properly. Obesity often contributes to the problem as excess fat cells displace insulin-receptor cells.

Since Type II appears most often in adults over the age of 40, this form may evolve from a gradual slowing of insulin production within the pancreas. In addition, other disorders of the endocrine system (glands that secrete hormones into the bloodstream) may cause hormonal imbalances that disturb insulin-sugar regulation.

185

Research shows that people who have Type II diabetes in their families have a greater tendency to acquire the condition. Women are more likely to be affected, but chances of developing Type II for all adults doubles with every decade past 40 years.

In some women, pregnancy triggers diabetes. The disease usually subsides after childbirth. However, women who show signs of diabetes during pregnancy and deliver babies weighing over ten pounds have a greater risk of diabetes later in life.

SYMPTOMS

Symptoms of Type I diabetes are excessive thirst and urination, fatigue, altered vision, fainting, irritability, and slow-healing cuts and bruises. Weight loss may occur despite constant hunger and voracious eating.

The same symptoms may signal Type II diabetes, or no symptoms may show at all. Doctors frequently detect this form when they perform routine urine examinations or tests for other problems.

DIAGNOSIS

Should no symptoms be obvious, doctors can diagnose diabetes by analysing blood and urine samples for elevated sugar concentrations. They may also test blood for extra insulin and urine for excess ketones. Ketones are the end products of breaking down fat for energy. Since people with diabetes do not use sugar normally, their bodies burn fat for fuel and eliminate the ketone end-products in the urine.

COMPLICATIONS

Even though patients with diabetes can usually control the condition, untreated diabetes can lead to serious complications. Extremely high blood sugar levels place great strain on other organs. Diabetes may trigger atherosclerosis, hardening and narrowing of arteries that carry blood throughout the body. Insufficient blood supply contributes to heart attack; stroke; kidney disease; eye disorders, such as retinopathy; impotence; death of tissue due to inadequate blood circulation; gangrene; and even death.

TREATMENT

Both forms of diabetes mellitus require a treatment plan that maintains normal steady blood glucose levels. Once blood sugar levels are under control with insulin injections, diet, or medication, a person with diabetes can usually lead a normal life.

Type I, or insulin-dependent, diabetes requires injections of insulin to regulate blood sugar levels evenly all day. If blood glucose concentrations rise, the body may signal an imbalance by displaying symptoms of weakness, fatigue and thirst. These symptoms mean that increased insulin is needed. However, if blood sugar levels become too low, an insulin reaction sets in, causing dizziness, hunger, fatigue, headache, sweating, trembling, and – in severe cases – unconsciousness. A quick remedy for this problem is to eat simple sugar, such as sweets or biscuits.

Ideally, a doctor can prevent these fluctuations of sugar levels by coordinating the type and timing of insulin injections with meal content and energy output. A special diet is important to balance daily insulin injections. Young children with diabetes, in particular, need sufficient calories to grow and develop normally. Insulin requirements for persons with Type I diabetes differ widely among individuals. Some patients may maintain balanced blood sugar levels with one insulin injection taken before breakfast. Other patients may require several insulin injections per day. Furthermore, insulin requirements may change as the patient grows older, undergoes surgery, becomes pregnant, or develops another unrelated illness.

Most people with Type II, or insulin-independent, diabetes can regulate their condition by proper diet. Sometimes, oral antidiabetic drugs, which work by stimulating the pancreas to produce more insulin or to make the body more sensitive to its effects, may be prescribed.

A controlled diet is critical for diabetes control. Overweight individuals need to lose weight. Thereafter, emphasis is on eating balanced meals that will sustain recommended weight. Fats need to be limited to reduce chances of atherosclerosis, and the diet should be low in simple sugars. The diet should include plenty of fibrous roughage, such as is contained in fruits, vegetables, and whole grains; fibre in the diet has been shown to reduce or slow sugar absorption in the digestive tract. Your doctor can provide a medically approved diet plan with food exchanges that allow flexibility with regular family meals and dietary needs.

With either type of diabetes, follow-up is important to plan diet, determine changes in insulin dosage, and re-test blood and urine for blood sugar levels. Increasingly, diabetics are taking control of their own health by performing blood and urine tests at home, and adjusting their insulin accordingly. Careful control of blood sugar levels can enable a person with diabetes to lead a normal life.

DIVERTICULITIS

Diverticulitis is the inflammation and/or infection of little sacs or pouches (diverticula) that have ballooned out through the walls of the colon (large intestine). The pouches form when the inner lining of the colon is forced under pressure through weaker spots in the colon's muscular layer. The existence of the pouches (as a condition, not a disease) is referred to as diverticulosis.

Diverticulosis may be present in about one third of the people over 60, and both its incidence and the frequency of complications increase with age.

CAUSES
One theory as to the cause of diverticulosis is that abnormal movement of the colon (possibly because of too little bulk in the diet) produces intense pressure that forces intestinal lining through the weak spots in the muscular layer. Most people with simple diverticulosis have no symptoms. Occasionally, however, a pouch next to a blood vessel may ulcerate, causing it to bleed. If the vessel is an artery, severe bleeding can result, seen as bleeding from the anus. Shock and possible death may result if the condition is not treated.

It has been estimated that about one-fifth to a quarter of

the people with diverticulosis may develop the symptoms of diverticulitis. Diverticulitis develops when a mass of hardened waste matter (called a faecalith) forms in a pouch and reduces the blood supply to the thin walls of the pouch (by means of pressure against the wall), making them more liable to infection by the bacteria of the colon. The inflammation that follows can lead to perforation, abscess (an enclosed sac of pus around the perforation), or infection of the lining of the abdominal cavity (peritonitis). Not infrequently, the inflamed section of bowel attaches to the urinary bladder or vagina, burrowing out from the colon to create a fistula (channel) that leaks infection into the other organ. Repeated inflammation can cause thickening of the wall of the colon, narrowing the colon and causing partial or sometimes total obstruction.

SYMPTOMS
Symptoms include intermittent cramping pains and tenderness, usually in the lower left abdomen but sometimes in other areas of the lower abdomen in which case the pains may resemble those of appendicitis. Pain that worsens during urination may indicate that the inflamed colon is attached to the bladder. Stool (faeces) and/or air in the urine may indicate a colon-to-bladder fistula. Constipation or constipation alternating with diarrhoea is common. Fever is usually present with acute attacks.

DIAGNOSIS
The diagnosis of diverticulitis usually is made if there is a history of pain in the left lower quadrant (quarter) of the abdomen accompanied by fever and a change in bowel habits. A physical examination may reveal a mass in the left lower quadrant along with extreme tenderness. After the acute episode has subsided, the examining doctor may insert a proctoscope (a lighted tube) through the anus and up the colon to be sure that there is no evidence of cancer that might be causing the symptoms. A barium (X-ray contrast fluid) enema and X-ray is usually done to further rule out cancer of the colon and to locate diverticula, obstructions, and fistulas.

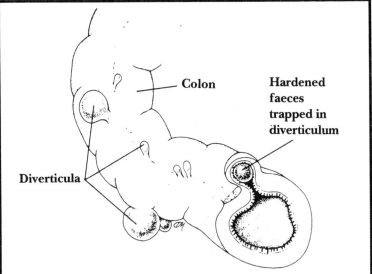

Colon

Hardened faeces trapped in diverticulum

Diverticula

Diverticulitis is the inflammation of the small pouches (diverticula) that have ballooned out from the colon wall due to the condition called diverticulosis. The inflammation often develops when a mass of hardened waste material (faeces) becomes trapped in a diverticulum, reducing the blood supply to the pouch wall and making it more susceptible to infection from bacteria in the colon.

TREATMENT

Treatment of severe diverticulitis begins with bed rest in a hospital and intravenous (in the vein) feeding with nothing by mouth (to give the intestine a rest). Antibiotics are given if there is fever or other evidence of an infection. If peritonitis (inflammation and/or infection of the lining of the abdominal cavity) develops, it may be necessary to operate. The inflamed section of the colon may simply be cut out and the remaining sections joined, or, more often, a temporary colostomy (in which the colon empties through an opening in the abdominal wall to the outside) may be necessary. Later, after all inflammation and infection has subsided, this is reconnected to the remaining colon or rectum.

PREVENTION

A diet with plenty of bulk appears to be a way to avoid

190

diverticulosis, the pouching that precedes diverticulitis. Those people who have developed diverticulosis should eat a relatively high-fibre diet. Supplements, such as Regulan, Fybogel or just ground bran, which increase bulk, may be recommended to move the stool through the colon at a normal rate.

GALL-STONES

Gall-stones are hardened masses that consist mainly of cholesterol, a substance regularly found in animal fats, blood, bile (fluid produced in the liver and stored in the gall bladder that is required for fat absorption in the small intestine), the liver, and other tissues. The stones form in the gall bladder or in the bile duct leading from the gall bladder into the small intestine, where food is digested and nutrients absorbed into the blood.

CAUSES
When bile contains excessive amounts of cholesterol in comparison to other ingredients, the unnecessary cholesterol separates from the solution and forms stone-like masses. Unfortunately, these stones cannot be prevented by controlling cholesterol intake in the diet. Cholesterol from food passes into the blood, and there is no relationship between cholesterol levels in the blood and cholesterol levels in the bile.

In addition to concentrated bile and bile salts, several other factors contribute to the formation of gall-stones. Eating too much fat, infection, liver disease, and forms of anaemia – such as sickle-cell anaemia – can lead to gall-stones.

Pregnancy, obesity, or diabetes can also increase the risk of gall-stones. Overweight people who frequently lose and gain large amounts of weight seem more susceptible to gall-stones, as do women who have had two or more children. Although reasons are unclear, twice as many women as men over age 40 develop gall-stones.

SYMPTOMS

By themselves, gall-stones often produce no signs of disease. About half the people with gall-stones have no symptoms. Symptoms that do appear are usually chronic (long-term) in nature, causing discomfort and pain in the upper abdomen, indigestion, nausea, and intolerance of fatty foods. Sometimes stones pass through the bile duct into the intestines to be excreted naturally.

However, symptoms can occur if the stones lodge in the bile duct. In an acute attack, called biliary colic, a sharp pain often on the right side of the upper abdomen may travel to the back and under the right shoulder blade. Frequently, the pain develops suddenly after a meal and leads to vomiting, and possibly jaundice (yellowing of the skin and whites of the eyes caused by excess bile pigment). These symptoms occur after a stone that was previously free-floating in the gall bladder becomes trapped in the bile duct.

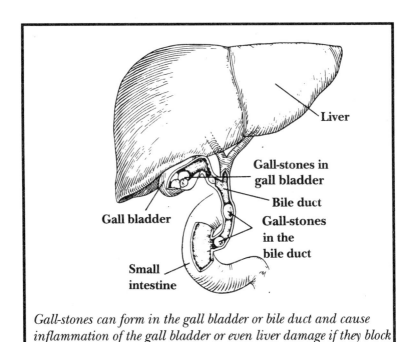

Gall-stones can form in the gall bladder or bile duct and cause inflammation of the gall bladder or even liver damage if they block the flow of bile from the gall bladder to the small intestine.

COMPLICATIONS

Serious complications of liver damage or jaundice may develop if stones block the flow of bile. Pressure from the stones may also cause inflammation and damage to nearby organs.

When gall-stones remain in the gall bladder, the organ may become inflamed with a condition called cholecystitis, which causes severe pain 30 to 60 minutes after eating.

DIAGNOSIS

Gall-stones that show no symptoms may be detected by an X-ray of the gall bladder called a cholecystogram. A cholecystogram is taken after the patient swallows a tablet containing dye which outlines the gall bladder and any stones that may be present. Nowadays most doctors use ultrasound rather than X-ray; ultrasound is a procedure in which sound waves bounce off internal body organs and construct a visual image.

TREATMENT

For acute attacks of gall-stones with severe and prolonged symptoms, doctors recommend a cholecystectomy (surgical removal of the gall bladder). This treatment is one of the most common forms of abdominal surgery, since the gall bladder is not necessary to maintain life. However, few doctors would normally suggest removing a gall bladder containing stones that is not causing symptoms.

Patients who are too old or unwell for surgery may benefit from drugs to dissolve gall-stones, although they don't work for everyone. More recently doctors have started to use high intensity sound shock waves to break gall-stones into fragments that will pass on their own. And new techniques mean that the operation to remove the gall bladder can often be done entirely through a laparoscope – a thin telescope – with only a tiny cut in the abdomen.

GASTROENTERITIS

Gastroenteritis is an inflammation of the lining of the stomach and the intestine.

CAUSES
Gastroenteritis can be caused by bacteria or viruses; by allergic reactions to certain foods or to certain drinks; by infectious diseases, such as typhoid fever or influenza; by food poisoning; by overconsumption of alcohol; or by certain drugs.

SYMPTOMS
Symptoms include headache, nausea, vomiting, diarrhoea, and pains in the stomach and the intestine. Often, the individual will feel that gas is 'caught' in certain portions of the intestine. On occasions, the intestines will seem to cramp, producing severe pain.

DIAGNOSIS
The first task in treating gastroenteritis is to identify the cause or causes of the inflammation. Usually, with a sudden and short-lived bout of infection, the doctor will assume that one of the common viruses is to blame and no tests are necessary. Otherwise blood tests or stool cultures for viruses or bacteria may be done.

TREATMENT
A bout of gastroenteritis will usually settle in a few days without treatment, although diarrhoea may persist for a week or 10 days. If symptoms haven't settled by then see your doctor.

The greatest danger is fluid loss, especially in the elderly or young children. The most important part of treatment is to replace this fluid, by small but frequent drinks. Powders containing salt and sugar mixtures, available from chemists, mix with water to produce a drink that is readily absorbed by the damaged bowel.

Anti-diarrhoea drugs can help symptoms if you have to work

or travel, but they don't clear up the illness any more quickly and may even prolong it. Antibiotics may make things worse too, unless gastroenteritis is caused by particular bacteria.

PREVENTION

Maintaining a clean kitchen, eating in restaurants where the kitchens are kept clean, washing fresh foods thoroughly, and cooking foods carefully, are all safeguards against bacterial and viral infections. Identification of allergy-causing foods and moderation in alcohol consumption also help prevent gastroenteritis if these are the causes of the problem.

HAEMORRHOIDS

Haemorrhoids, often called piles, are enlarged veins inside or just outside the anal canal, which is the opening at the end of the large intestine. As veins swell, they cause severe inflammation and discomfort.

CAUSES

In most cases, haemorrhoids are the result of individual toilet habits whereby some people postpone normal bowel functioning.

Habitual postponement of bowel movements can lead to loss of rectal function and undesirable straining during elimination. Straining irritates veins and slows the flow of blood, thereby contributing to swollen or inflamed veins. Postponing bowel movements may also cause stools retained in the bowels to lose moisture. When faeces become dry and hard, the added strain of constipation encourages haemorrhoids.

Diet plays a major role in the development of haemorrhoids. A diet containing a high proportion of refined foods, such as white flour and sugar, rather than foods with natural roughage, increases the likelihood of constipation and, therefore, the likelihood of haemorrhoids.

Another source of haemorrhoid irritation comes from pressure on the veins from diseases of the liver or heart or from a tumour. Pregnancy also contributes to the development of haemorrhoids because the enlarged uterus increases pressure on the veins. Moreover, prolonged pressure from pushing during labour and delivery can inflame the area. Although women appear to develop haemorrhoids during pregnancy, recent research suggests that they probably had the condition prior to pregnancy.

Haemorrhoids seem to be more prevalent in some families. However, this tendency has been attributed to similar dietary and personal habits.

SYMPTOMS

Haemorrhoids may take years to develop and often result in irritating symptoms. The first signs of haemorrhoids include itching and some discomfort during and after bowel movements. Continued straining during elimination will eventually produce slight swelling of the lining of the anal canal. This swelling may not be noticed until hard stools scrape the anal lining and cause slight bleeding – an early clue that a haemorrhoid may have developed.

With prolonged straining, a portion of the anal canal may jut out of the anus during a bowel movement. At this stage, the elastic connective tissue is still strong enough to pull the haemorrhoid back into the anal canal unassisted, so the individual may not notice the growing problem. However, with persistent pressure, the protruding tissue may remain outside the anus after a bowel movement and need to be manually returned to the anal canal. Once outside the anal canal, the haemorrhoid often creates a dull aching sensation.

A more involved problem develops when the haemorrhoid is difficult or impossible to return, and permanent swelling at the anal opening interferes with elimination. Then the patient may postpone bowel movements in an effort to avoid pain. Instead of helping, this intensifies the problem, because it leads to constipation.

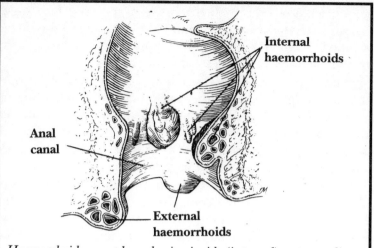

Internal
haemorrhoids

Anal
canal

External
haemorrhoids

Haemorrhoids are enlarged veins inside (internal) or protruding
from (external) the anal canal. These swollen veins cause itching
and pain which may be accompanied by bleeding.

DIAGNOSIS

To diagnose a haemorrhoid, the doctor inspects the anal
canal, often with special instruments. A proctoscope (short,
lighted tube) inserted into the anus can reveal the condition
of the rectal lining. A sigmoidoscope, which is a longer instrument, shows a view of the inner area of the colon.

TREATMENT

Painful haemorrhoids can be treated at home by applying
cold water compresses directly to the anal area for five to ten
minutes until pain is relieved. Some people reduce pain by
taking hot baths. Over-the-counter preparations cannot cure
haemorrhoids, but they can relieve itching and swelling.
Should symptoms worsen after application of any remedy, its
use should be suspended and a doctor consulted. Chemicals
in these preparations may produce an allergic reaction. Non-
irritating laxatives may also be occasionally useful in softening
stools and easing bowel movements.

In the early stages of haemorrhoid development, adjustment of personal habits may prevent progression of the

197

condition. A bowel movement should never be delayed, once the urge is felt. During bowel movements, straining should be avoided. A diet including plenty of roughage – natural grains, fresh fruits, and vegetables – also soften stools.

For severe cases of haemorrhoids, a doctor may recommend a surgical procedure called haemorrhoidectomy to remove dilated portions of the affected veins and tie off the remaining parts of the vein. Less severe cases are often treated by injecting a substance such as phenol into the haemorrhoids, to make them shrink and shrivel.

Another technique used to eliminate internal haemorrhoids is rubber band ligation. Here, the doctor ties off the haemorrhoids blood supply with a special instrument. This procedure causes the haemorrhoid to die and drop off within three to nine days. Once the haemorrhoid dies, brief spotting of blood and minor itching may occur.

HEPATITIS

Hepatitis is a viral infection of the liver that is characterised by jaundice, a yellowing of the skin and whites of the eyes.

CAUSES AND TYPES

The disease is caused by several viruses, but the most common virus strains of hepatitis are hepatitis A, or infectious hepatitis, and hepatitis B, or serum hepatitis. A third virus, hepatitis C, has recently been discovered and is the commonest cause of hepatitis following a blood transfusion in this country.

All strains enter the body as minute organisms and attack cells in the liver. Hepatitis A passes through the digestive tract and is transmitted from person to person by contaminated food or water or through the stools of an infected person. This form may occur as epidemics in places where sanitation is poor and sewage contaminated. Incubation, the time between exposure to the disease and the appearance of symptoms, is between 14 to 40 days. Sometimes, hepatitis A is so mild that symptoms never appear, but the infected person can still transmit the disease as a carrier of infection.

With hepatitis B, the virus enters the bloodstream, either from transfusion of contaminated blood or from contaminated needles, especially among drug users. Hepatitis B begins more gradually than does hepatitis A, so the disease may be present 40 to 180 days before the onset of symptoms. In addition, the virus can live in almost all body fluids, including saliva, semen, urine, and tears. This allows hepatitis B to be transmitted by sexual contact or by more casual contact such as sharing toothbrushes or razors.

Hepatitis may also result as a complication of the viral infection called infectious mononucleosis (glandular fever).

SYMPTOMS

Early signs of hepatitis are general fatigue, joint and muscle pain, and loss of appetite. Nausea, vomiting, and diarrhoea or constipation may follow, with a low-grade fever of 39°C or less. As the disease develops, the liver enlarges and becomes tender. Chills, weight loss, and distaste for smoking appear along with the characteristic jaundice. Jaundice results from an accumulation of yellow bile pigment in the blood that turns the skin and whites of the eyes yellow.

In hepatitis A, the disappearance of jaundice generally signals the beginning of recovery. However, in hepatitis B, the virus may persist for years or the duration of a lifetime.

Any sudden rise in fever, extreme drowsiness, or severe prolonged pain requires immediate medical supervision to avoid permanent liver damage. Chronic, long-term hepatitis can lead to irreversible liver failure or cirrhosis.

DIAGNOSIS

To determine the extent and severity of hepatitis, a doctor analyses blood and urine specimens from the suspected hepatitis patient. If the disease has progressed, the patient may have yellow skin and soreness in the upper abdomen over the liver.

More severe chronic hepatitis may require a liver biopsy, in which a needle is inserted into the liver to obtain a sample of liver tissue. In this procedure, local anaesthetic is usually injected into the upper abdomen to eliminate discomfort from the test.

New blood tests can spot hepatitis B and identify carriers of the virus.

TREATMENT

Because hepatitis is caused by a virus, there is no cure. Even treatment is limited, especially for acute hepatitis. Once the virus attacks, recovery is usually up to the body's regular defence system.

To encourage the healing process, doctors advise patients to avoid all strenuous activity. Strict bed rest is more important during the acute phases of hepatitis. More serious cases may require hospitalisation to ensure inactivity. Some of these patients may also need an exchange blood transfusion to aid recovery if the body cannot overcome contamination by itself. In addition, all hepatitis patients must avoid alcoholic beverages, because processing alcohol puts a tremendous strain on the liver.

PREVENTION

People exposed to hepatitis can prevent or minimise the disease by obtaining an injection of gamma globulin, a disease-fighting substance in the blood. Gamma globulin usually defends against virus A and offers a modest protection against virus B. In either case, if hepatitis develops following an injection, gamma globulin seems to reduce symptoms.

Scientists have also developed new vaccines against hepatitis A and B. A vaccine is a preparation of the disease-causing agent that is introduced into the body to stimulate the body to produce antibodies whose job it is to fight the disease. For now, hepatitis B vaccine is only recommended for people who are in direct contact with hepatitis carriers, but the vaccine may eventually be recommended for more widespread use. Hepatitis A vaccine is recommended for travellers to countries where standards of hygiene don't match our own.

HERNIA

The term hernia refers to any abnormal protrusion of part of an organ or tissue(s) through the structures that normally contain it. In this condition, a weak spot or opening in a body wall allows part of the organ to bulge through. A hernia may develop in almost any part of the body; however, the most common sites are the abdominal and groin areas.

Although a hernia is often popularly called a 'rupture', this is a misleading description. Nothing is actually 'torn' or ruptured in a hernia. A hernia can be congenital (present at birth) or acquired; in the latter case, it is often the result of some stress or strain on the body wall involved.

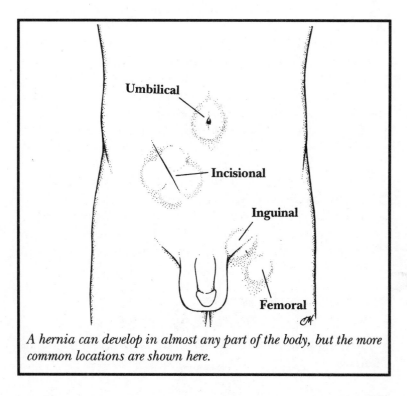

A hernia can develop in almost any part of the body, but the more common locations are shown here.

COMMON TYPES OF HERNIAS

Although there are literally as many types of hernias as there are sites or locations in the body, the following are some of the most common hernias:

- Umbilical hernia, protrusion of part of the intestine at the navel or umbilicus (seen mostly in infants).
- Inguinal hernia, a protrusion of a loop of intestine into the groin where the folds of abdominal flesh meet the thighs, often the result of increased pressure in the abdomen because of lifting, coughing, straining, or accidents (accounts for about 75 per cent of all common hernias).
- Scrotal hernia, an inguinal hernia that has passed into the scrotum, the bag of skin behind the penis that contains the testes.
- Femoral hernia, a protrusion of a loop of intestine into the femoral canal, which is a tubular passageway that carries nerves and blood vessels from the abdomen into the thigh (this type of hernia is more common in women than in men).
- Incisional hernia, a hernia that occurs after an operation at the site of the surgical incision; often this type of hernia is due to excessive strain on the healing tissue (excessive muscular effort, lifting, coughing, or extreme obesity, which puts pressure on a weakened area).
- Hiatus hernia (also called diaphragmatic hernia) occurs when a portion of the stomach protrudes above the diaphragm, the muscular wall separating the chest and abdominal cavities, into the chest. Normally, the oesophagus (the passageway from the throat to the stomach) passes through a tight muscular collar that prevents the stomach from squeezing up into the chest cavity. However, if the collar is too large or relaxes, a sliding hiatus hernia may occur.

CONDITIONS OF HERNIAS

Hernias can also be classified by their condition:

- Irreducible hernia, one that cannot be restored by manipulation.

- Reducible hernia, one that can be returned to 'normal' by manipulation.
- Incarcerated hernia, a hernia that cannot be reduced through treatment, but is not obstructed or strangulated.
- Strangulated hernia, one that is tightly constricted, cutting off the blood supply of the affected tissue.

SYMPTOMS
Because of the many different types of hernias, the symptoms will vary slightly depending on the cause and the body part(s) involved.

DIAGNOSIS
Diagnosis of a hernia can usually be made by thorough visual examination and by studying the patient's medical history and symptoms.

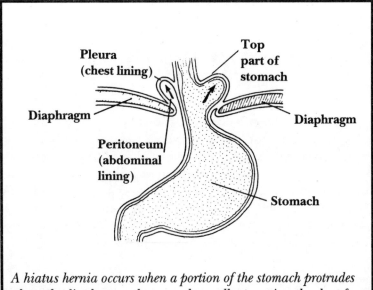

A hiatus hernia occurs when a portion of the stomach protrudes above the diaphragm, the muscular wall separating the chest from the abdomen.

TREATMENT

For small, non-strangulated or non-incarcerated hernias, various supports and trusses can sometimes offer temporary, symptomatic relief. However, the best treatment is surgical closure or repair of the structure through which the hernia protrudes. Surgical repair of a hernia is called herniorrhaphy. When the weakened area is very large, some strong synthetic material may be sewn over the defect to reinforce the weak area. Post-operative care is simple and involves protecting the patient from respiratory infections that would cause him/her to cough and sneeze, thus placing strain on the suture line. Recovery is usually quick and complete.

Treatment of hiatus hernia usually involves medication to counteract the effects of stomach acid, or to prevent acid escaping from the stomach into the gullet. This prevents heartburn, the usual symptom of a hiatus hernia.

PREVENTION

Avoiding strain or pressure on any body wall, especially those of the abdomen and groin area (in men), is the only real preventive measure against hernias.

JAUNDICE

Jaundice is a yellowish discolouration of the skin, whites of the eyes, mucous membranes, and other tissues of the body, and is caused by the abnormal accumulation of bile pigment (or bilirubin) in the blood. Bilirubin consists primarily of the haemoglobin of used red blood cells and is found in bile, a yellow-green fluid that aids in the digestion of fat. Bile is secreted by the liver, stored in the gall bladder, and discharged into the intestine when needed.

CAUSES

In many cases, jaundice occurs when bile is prevented by obstruction from being discharged into the intestine. The obstruction may be caused by gall stones, by tumours or, uncommonly, by parasites in the bile ducts. Jaundice may also be an accompanying sign of hepatitis, a disorder in which the inflamed or damaged liver cannot process the bilirubin it receives. Occasionally, jaundice appears if too many red blood cells are too rapidly destroyed, sometimes as a result of an anaemic condition, and the liver cannot accommodate the excess. In addition, jaundice is associated with, or symptomatic of, many other diseases in which the normal functioning of the liver is disrupted. These diseases include certain cancers and certain viral and parasitic infections. Over 50 per cent of full-term and 80 per cent of premature newborns show signs of jaundice by the second or third day after birth. In most of these cases, however, the condition is nothing to worry about and disappears in a week or so.

SYMPTOMS
When jaundice occurs, the liver usually has become enlarged and functions less effectively. Bowel movements may be clay-coloured, and urine can vary in hue from light yellow to a brownish green. Jaundiced skin ranges in colour from lemony yellow to dark olive green.

DIAGNOSIS
Routine blood testing will determine the origin of most cases of jaundice, but occasionally it may be necessary to observe the bile ducts, by means of an X-ray. Certain dyes injected into the blood will collect in the liver and bile ducts to show the point of obstruction on an X-ray. Other alternatives include ultrasound, in which sound waves bounce off internal body structures and form an image of them, and a CAT scan, a special technique that provides a cross-sectional picture of the area.

TREATMENT
If a back-up of bile is observed, surgery to eliminate the obstruction may be indicated. Otherwise, treatment will be determined by the nature of the cause of the jaundice.

PERIODONTAL DISEASE

Periodontal disease, or periodontitis, is a progressive deterioration of the gums and bones around the teeth.

CAUSES

One theory is that the condition begins with an accumulation of bacteria and food particles that lodge within tissues surrounding the teeth. These bacteria emit toxins (poisons) that cause gum tissues to swell, bleed, and erode.

Gingivitis, inflammation of the gums, is the first stage of periodontitis. Pyorrhea (running of pus), the second stage of periodontitis, results when the soft tissues are separated from the bone and teeth leading to 'pocket' formation. Pockets of bacteria and pus accumulate around the teeth leading to weakening of the fibres holding the teeth in their sockets as well as to destruction of the bone supporting the teeth. As the disease advances, teeth become loose and fall out. They may also move out of alignment with one another and cause problems with chewing.

SYMPTOMS

In the early stage of periodontal disease, gums become sore, red and slightly swollen. They may be sensitive to the touch and bleed when brushed or flossed. Pus in the gums around the teeth signals the beginning of the second disease stage. If pus remains in the gum tissue without draining, extreme pain and swelling can result.

DIAGNOSIS

A dentist diagnoses the beginning of periodontal disease by examining the swollen gums and the deposits of bacteria and plaque that accumulate around the teeth.

TREATMENT AND PREVENTION

Once detected, continued care of the mouth at home can help prevent extensive periodontal disease and reduce gum problems.

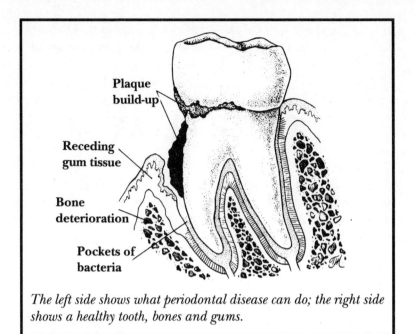

Plaque build-up

Receding gum tissue

Bone deterioration

Pockets of bacteria

The left side shows what periodontal disease can do; the right side shows a healthy tooth, bones and gums.

Oral hygiene to prevent gum disease is the same as treatment to prevent tooth decay. Ideally, the mouth needs to be cleaned after every meal. More realistically, a thorough cleansing before bed may minimise the chances of gum disease. Dentists suggest brushing teeth with a soft-bristled brush. Gentle movements within the crevices dislodge decay-causing material, while firm strokes over the teeth remove plaque.

Flossing is recommended to clear plaque from between teeth. After brushing and flossing, vigorously rinsing the mouth with mouthwash containing anti-microbials (substances that kill bacteria) can also help eliminate bacteria formation; but mouthwash alone cannot prevent plaque.

For self-checking, a dental mirror provides a view of the teeth and gums in the back of the mouth. Disclosing wafers, which when chewed discolour plaque, reveal any invisible film to be removed.

For advanced cases, a dentist may scrape the affected tissue pockets and apply antiseptics (germ-killers) every few months in an effort to kill the bacteria. Should this procedure fail to check the spread of the disease, surgery by a gum specialist may be needed to remove deep pockets in the gum. Once the bacteria are eliminated, good oral hygiene practices should control the disease.

TOOTH DECAY

Tooth decay (or dental cavities, or caries) is the gradual destruction and loss of minerals in the enamel (outer layer) and dentine (the bony second layer) of a portion of a tooth, which causes it to become soft, discoloured, and porous.

CAUSES
A combination of factors causes tooth decay. The actual destruction is probably done by bacteria and by-products of their metabolism such as acid. These bacteria feed on sugars and starches that cling to the teeth. They live and multiply to become dental plaque. The plaque is made up mainly of bacteria as well as sugars, starches and proteins, and builds up on dental surfaces, especially near the gums and in other hard-to-clean areas. Here the production of acid is concentrated. The plaque prevents the saliva from performing its natural protective function.

SYMPTOMS
When the cavity has progressed through the dentine or begins on the surface of an exposed root, the tooth becomes sensitive to touch and to rapid temperature changes. Sweet foods can cause pain as dissolved sugar enters the cavity. Bacteria may pass through tiny tubes in the dentine and inflame the pulp, which contains blood vessels and nervous tissue, producing toothache.

DIAGNOSIS
The cavity reveals itself to the examining dentist as a darkened area or as a softness that 'gives' when probed with a sharp instrument. It is also detected by X-rays.

TREATMENT

Cavities are treated by drilling out the decayed material and replacing it with a filling. In front teeth, where appearance is important, the filling may be of porcelain cement or a plastic resin (which is also used to fill pits and tiny cracks in the enamel). In other teeth the filling is usually silver-coloured or, if more extensive restoration is required, an alloy of gold, which is the most durable material. Tooth-coloured fillings of composite resin are also available, although not usually on the NHS.

Where a tooth is badly damaged with involvement of the root canal, the dentist removes all decay, fills the cavity and root canal with cement, then grinds and tapers the outer surfaces and covers them with what is known as a crown. On teeth toward the front, the crown is overlaid with porcelain or is made of tooth-coloured material to provide a natural appearance.

PREVENTION

To prevent decay, teeth should be cleaned for at least a couple of minutes daily with a medium nylon brush, preferably after each meal, to remove food particles and plaque. Equally important is the use of dental floss to remove debris between the teeth. Avoiding sweet, sticky foods between meals and brushing shortly after eating them, will also help prevent decay.

A child's teeth will be more resistant to decay if the child drinks water containing the proper amount of fluoride in the first 12 years while the teeth are developing. If the water supply is not fluoridated, a supplement containing fluoride can be taken daily. Adults and children alike can benefit by using a fluoride-containing toothpaste, although children using fluoride toothpaste shouldn't use fluoride drops as well.

Regular visits to your dentist's hygienist will help to ensure that you are looking after your teeth correctly. Make sure you have regular check-ups every 6 to 12 months.

ULCER

An ulcer is an open sore or erosion on the surface of an organ or tissue. The most common ulcers erupt in the digestive tract, in which case they are known as peptic ulcers. Peptic ulcers can appear in the lining of the oesophagus (tube leading to the stomach), stomach, or duodenum (beginning of the small intestine).

CAUSES
Although the cause of a peptic ulcer is unconfirmed, scientists believe that the more common duodenal ulcers may result from excessive amounts of digestive juices produced by the stomach. The stomach may increase acidic secretions after coffee, alcohol, aspirin and other painkillers are consumed, or after cigarettes are smoked. Therefore, these substances are thought to contribute to ulcers.

The less common stomach ulcers may be due to an inherent weakness in the wall of the stomach. Recent studies suggest that helicobacter, a bacterium that can live in the stomach may be an important cause of this weakness.

Emotional stress may play a role in ulcer development. However, doctors distinguish between stress as a factor by itself, and the way certain people deal with stress that would make them susceptible to ulcers.

Heredity plays an important role in contributing to ulcers since people who have a history of ulcers in their family seem to have a greater likelihood of acquiring the condition. Furthermore, for unknown reasons, people with Type O blood are more likely to develop ulcers. In addition, liver disease, rheumatoid arthritis (inflammation of connective tissue), and emphysema (over-inflation of the lungs' air sacs) may increase vulnerability to ulcers.

SYMPTOMS
Ulcers can produce mild symptoms resembling heartburn or indigestion, or severe pain radiating throughout the upper

portion of the body. The most common discomfort of ulcers is a burning in the abdomen above the navel that may feel like hunger pangs. Pain comes about 30 to 120 minutes after eating or in the middle of the night when the stomach is empty. At this time, the stomach's acidic juices are more apt to irritate the unprotected nerve endings in the exposed ulcer. Usually, pain subsides after eating or drinking something or taking an antacid to neutralise stomach acid.

Some people experience nausea, vomiting, and constipation. Blood in faeces (discolouring them black), blood in vomit, extreme weakness, fainting, and excessive thirst are all signs of internal bleeding, and may appear with more advanced ulcers.

While ulcers are not always life-threatening, they can cause serious damage if left untreated. Ulcers may corrode nearby blood vessels and cause internal seepage of blood or massive internal bleeding (haemorrhage). A perforated ulcer may penetrate an adjoining organ, causing infection. In addition, scar tissue growing around the ulcer may lead to an intestinal obstruction.

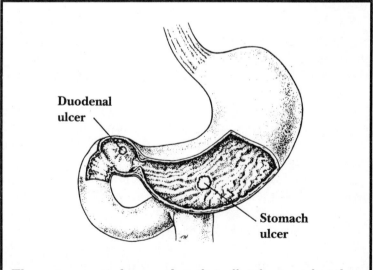

The most common ulcers are those that affect the stomach or the duodenum, the beginning section of the small intestine.

211

DIAGNOSIS

Until recently, doctors used to diagnose peptic ulcers primarily by X-ray. The patient swallows barium, a chalky substance, and stands in front of a fluorescent screen. As the X-ray tube moves down from the shoulder, the barium shows an opaque outline of the digestive tract that allows the doctor a view of any abnormalities.

Nowadays the doctor is more likely to use a gastroscope (long, flexible lighted tube) inserted through the mouth and down the oesophagus to see the ulcer. Stomach ulcers require a gastroscopic examination and a biopsy (removal of tissue sample for analysis) to confirm that the ulcer is not actually a cancer showing up as an ulcer on the X-ray.

TREATMENT

Treatment for ulcers involves relieving the irritation so healing progresses naturally. Over-the-counter antacids counteract stomach acid and relieve symptoms, but they can cause complications. For example, sodium bicarbonate, a primary antacid ingredient, contains large amounts of sodium (salt) that can aggravate kidney disease or high blood pressure.

For more problematic ulcers, a doctor may prescribe other preparations to promote healing. Recently combinations of antibiotics and drugs containing bismuth have been increasingly used. These work against stomach bacteria called helicobacter, which are now thought to be the cause of many stomach ulcers. Other drugs may form a protective coating against the acid in the stomach (for example sucralfate and carbenoxalone) or inhibit gastric acid secretion (for example cimetidine and ranitidine).

Nowadays a bland diet is unnecessary for ulcer management. Most doctors suggest avoiding only those foods known to cause stomach distress.

The effect of milk on ulcers is also questionable. Its neutralising action on stomach acid is mild and temporary at best. Nevertheless, people who substitute milk for alcohol or caffeine are less likely to irritate their ulcers.

Most ulcers heal within two to six weeks after treatment

begins. To prevent recurrence, patients should still refrain from cigarettes, caffeine, alcohol, or other agents that would stimulate stomach acid production or irritate the digestive tract lining.

When drug therapy and diet cannot cure an ulcer, surgical removal may be necessary. Surgery follows repeated ulcers or ulcers that are life-threatening, such as perforated ulcers. Sometimes, surgeons remove a portion of the stomach and parts of the vagus nerve (which controls digestive secretions) to reduce stomach acid production. Usually, ulcers do not reappear after surgery.

Index

Figures in italics refer to captions